SPA LIVING

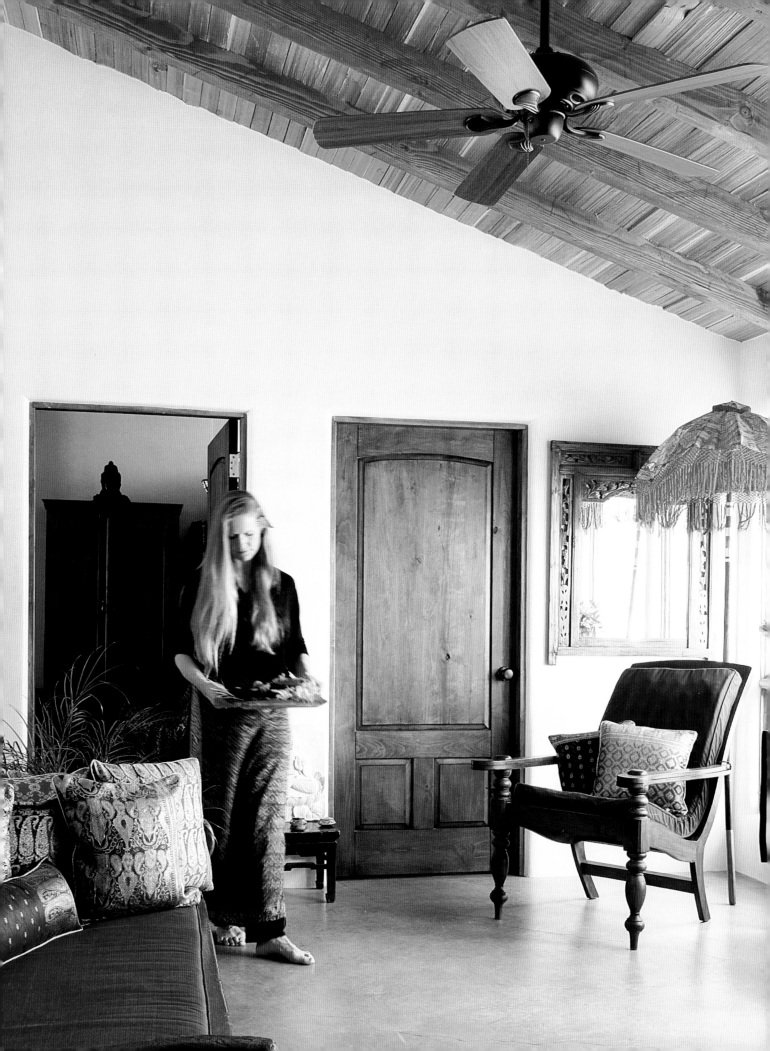

SPALIVING

IDEAS, TIPS & RECIPES FOR REVITALIZING BODY-MIND-SPIRIT

SUNAMITA LIM

Principal Photographer Kim Kurian

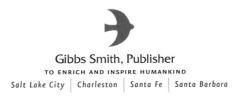

Gibbs Smith, Publisher
TO ENRICH AND INSPIRE HUMANKIND

Salt Lake City | Charleston | Santa Fe | Santa Barbara

First Edition
11 10 09 08 07   5 4 3 2 1

Text © 2007 Sunamita Lim
Photographs © 2007 as noted throughout and on page 189

Published by
Gibbs Smith, Publisher
P.O. Box 667
Layton, Utah 84041

Orders: 1.800.835.4993
www.gibbs-smith.com

Designed by m:GraphicDesign / Maralee Oleson
Printed and bound in China
Library of Congress Cataloging-in-Publication Data

Lim, Sunamita.
  Spa living : ideas, tips, and recipes for revitalizing body-mind-
spirit /
Sunamita Lim. — 1st ed.
     p. cm.
  Includes bibliographical references and index.
  ISBN-13: 978-1-4236-0102-9
  ISBN-10: 1-4236-0102-5
  1. Beauty, Personal. 2. Therapeutics, Physiological. 3. Health
resorts. I. Title.

RA776.98.L56 2007
613'.122—dc22
                                        2007015599

previous: Carolyn Lee, owner of Absolute
Nirvana Spa, in Santa Fe, New Mexico,
welcomes spa guests.

facing: An elegant bathroom detail garners
a second look at Cal-a-Vie. (Courtesy
photo)

Dedicated to seekers of Radiant Beauty
and Good Health, who revel in the
Soul's own True Light.

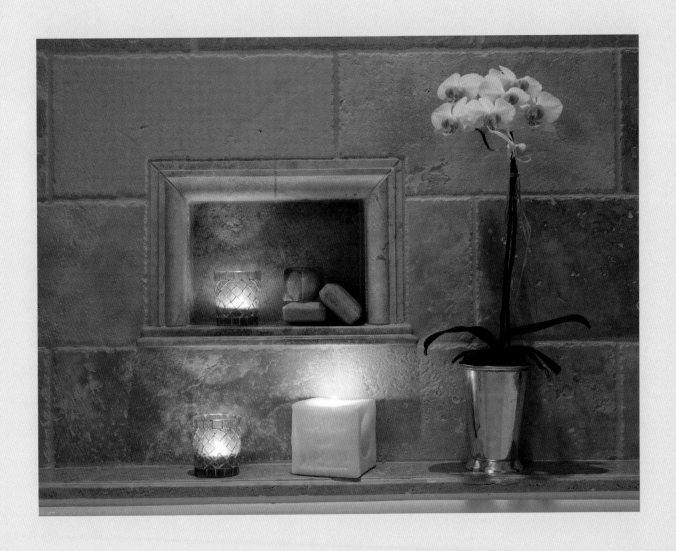

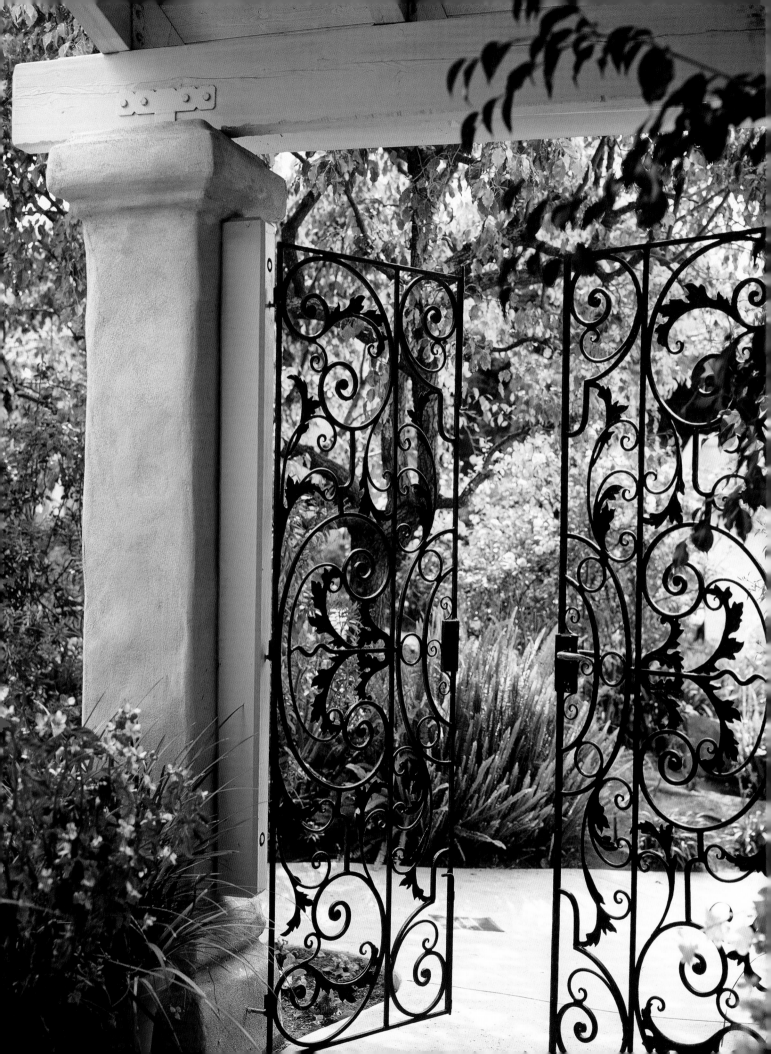

CONTENTS

An inviting entry to Cal-a-Vie's garden
from the sumptuous Bath House.
(Courtesy photo)

FOREWORD

With the questing spirit of a true pilgrim, Sunamita Lim recounts her tour of the spa world's inner and outer beauty. She enthusiastically visits many of the world's best destination spas and delves into their great appeal, from seeking serenity to joining in high-energy activities to enjoying delicious foods, as well as experiencing equally "delicious" and soothing treatments.

Today, the appeal of destination spas seems unquestionable as you leaf through this book. Yet it wasn't always so. When my husband, Edmond, and I started Rancho La Puerta in 1940, we had a core group of loyal guests who had been to Edmond's "health camps" before, or had read his many books on living the healthier, simpler life. The outside world, however, considered us a cult because of our then-unfathomable recommendations to eat foods grown without pesticides or fertilizers, exercise daily, find a mind/body/spirit balance, never smoke, avoid drinking distilled spirits, never stop learning and challenging the intellect, and other paradigms now considered the basic tenets of living a healthy, longer life.

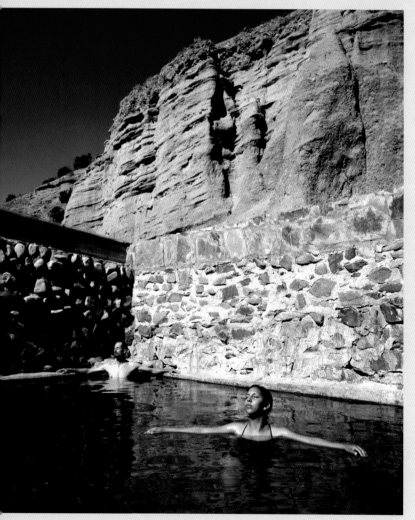

It pleases me that the days of the media and other pundits calling spas "fat farms" are long behind us. Spas are not about deprivation. Today's guests wish to enjoy the fullness of nature, the camaraderie of new friends, and a glorious feeling of wellness. They also seek their future, for any great spa provides the inspiration and means with which to reinvent the next exciting phase of one's life.

In the future, destination spas will have a new mission which I believe is vital to our society's well-being. Productivity and the fast life have become society's relentless mantra. Many people have given up pleasure, leisure, family, and community. We must slow down, especially in the way we approach our food. Today's spas, along with the international organization Slow Food, advocate a return to the dining ritual, a prolonging of the pleasure. It begins on the farm, in the market, and is multiplied by every step made in the kitchen . . . all culminating in the joy of being with family and friends gathered at the table.

Exercise is not enough. The other half of good health is food, nutrition, nourishment, and nurturing—the preconditions to survival.

If the spa experience is to be described in a single word, one might select *pleasure*—deep, abiding pleasure. May the pleasure begin now, as you enjoy Sunamita Lim's inspiring and informative tour of the spa world.

—Deborah Szekely, Founder, Rancho La Puerta (1940)
and the Golden Door (1958)

facing: Soaking in sun and minerals at Ojo Caliente, New Mexico. (Courtesy photo)

The Provençal-style entrance to Cal-a-Vie's Fitness Center provides an unexpected counterpoint to its gym facilities. (Courtesy photo)

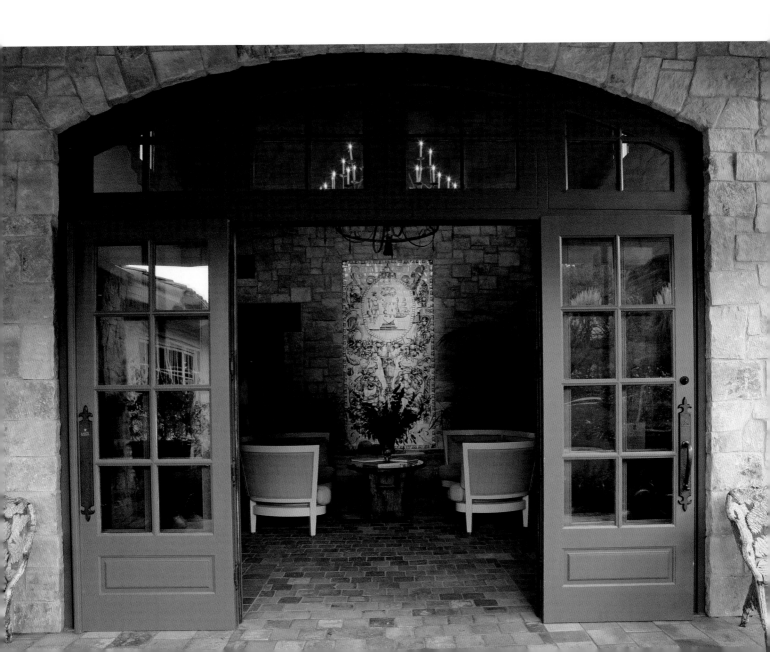

ACKNOWLEDGMENTS

A stone lodge purifies peaceably at Sunrise Springs, Santa Fe.

facing: The women's outdoor hot tub taps into a rustic setting at Ten Thousand Waves Japanese Spa and Retreat, Santa Fe, New Mexico.

The soothing, silky touch of facials and salubrious euphoria from expert massage sessions lead me to offer heartfelt gratitude first to these dedicated professionals. They offer a different kind of nurturing—while advocating natural beauty for good health.

Many thanks also go to the doyenne of the modern spa, Deborah Szekely, for writing the foreword to this book. Deborah and her late husband, Edmond, pioneered the American destination spa movement with Rancho La Puerta, south of San Diego in Tecate, Mexico, in 1940. In 1958, Deborah founded the elegant spa sanctuary, Golden Door, in Escondido, California.

From day spas to destination spas, which require a minimum of three-night stays, the sense of personal enhancement and satisfaction is deeply felt by guests. My sincere appreciation

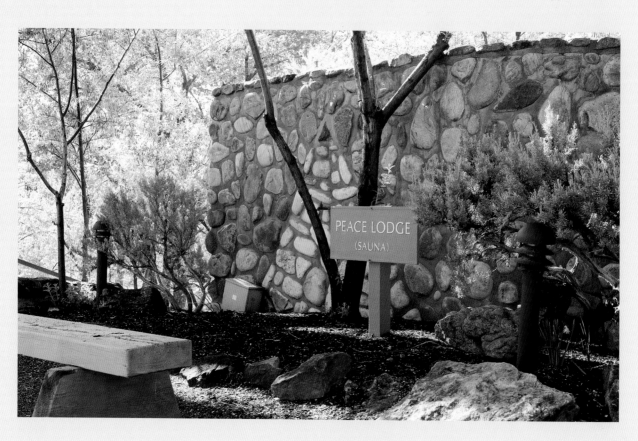

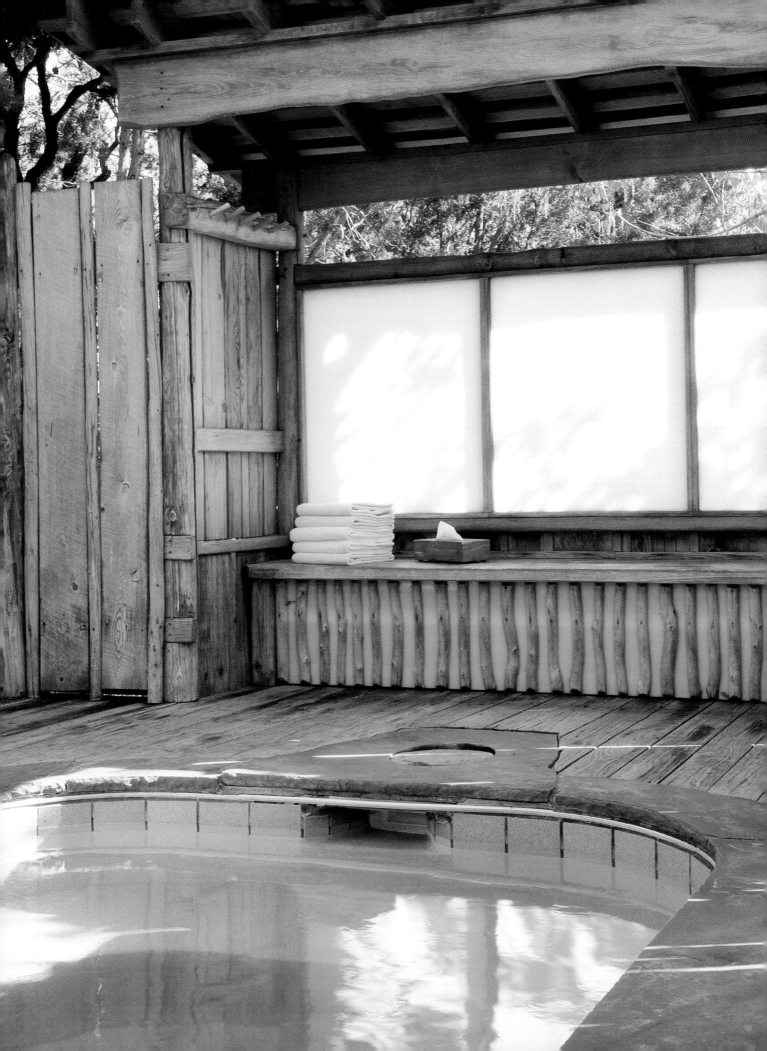

goes to the following spas, which have been generous with their hospitality.

The diverse voices of spa directors, managers, aestheticians, and therapists are reflected in their words on radiant beauty that these knowledgeable individuals have kindly shared in my quest to uncover a keener awareness of the concept of "beauty."

In addition to full spa listings in the Resources section at the back of this book, I would like to list them here too.

Day spas include: Absolute Nirvana; Avanyu; BODY; Chopra Center New York; Cornelia Day Spa & Resort; El Monte Sagrado; Four Seasons Hotel Spas in New York City, Philadelphia, and Washington, D.C.; God's Beauty; Ihilani; Mandarin Oriental in New York and Washington, D.C.; Nidah; Nob Hill; Ojo Caliente; Olympus; Ritz-Carlton New York; Safety Harbor; Salish Lodge; ShaNah; SpaHalekulani; SpaOlakino; SpaTerre; Spa Vitale; Tamaya Mist; Ten Thousand Waves; Terme di Aroma; and The Westin at Times Square in New York City.

Destination spas include: Cal-a-Vie, Golden Door, and Rancho La Puerta.

Finally, no book project is complete without sterling efforts from members of the editorial team. They include editorial director Suzanne Taylor, managing editor Madge Baird, senior editor Jennifer Grillone, editor Hollie Keith, designer Maralee Oleson, and visual asset manager Lety Le Bleu. And, a big "thank-you" to everyone at Gibbs Smith, Publisher, for their hard work in bringing to light another informative and elegant lifestyle book.

—Sunamita Lim
Santa Fe, New Mexico

facing: Softly flowing water and natural light define an inviting spa relaxation area. (Courtesy, La Posada de Santa Fe Resort & Spa)

A cooling touch of the tropics refreshes visually at SpaOlakino, Honolulu. (Courtesy photo)

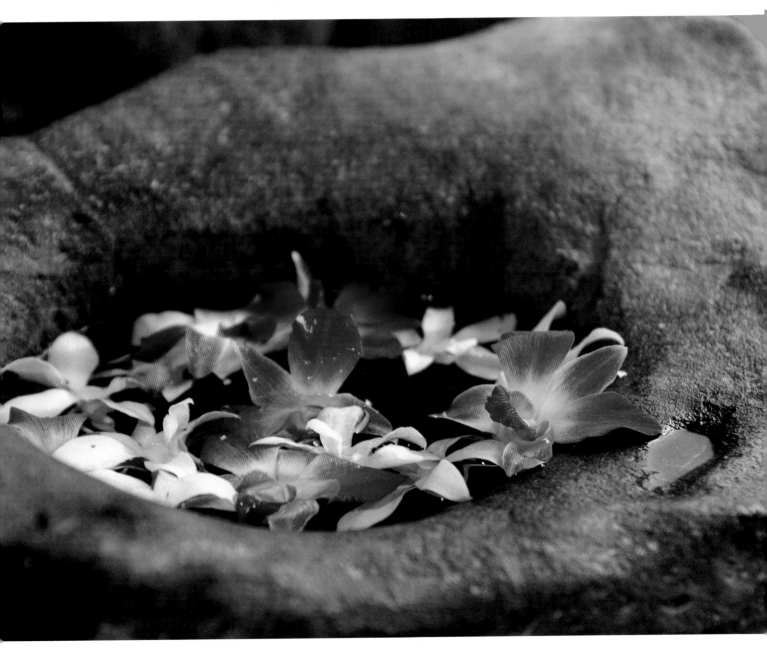

INTRODUCTION

A cheerful mind

Has always been

A perfect guide

To a healthy body.

—Sri Chinmoy, Meditation Master and Powerlifter

In writing this introduction, I am humbled and grateful to see Light at the end of a decade-long odyssey to regain *hozho*, or "walking in beauty," as the Navajos call it. I'm enjoying a sense of well-being at rediscovering myself in deeper ways, thanks to taking to the waters and with spa treatments.

It's a quiet joy grounded in love of, and faith in, the Divine—emotions similar to those when, as a kid, I played with exuberance and abandon at the playground, but much deeper.

And, it is a privilege to share my story in hopes of inspiring others to start looking within—to prevent, mitigate, and/or heal life-changing situations we all face at various times on Life's myriad adventurous journeys.

In June 1997, I'd been packing and excited about going on the road for a week with the global relay World Harmony Run (www.worldharmonyrun.org). Then, from out of the blue, a bolt of burning energy tore through my left arm as I was loading up my car—making me wonder if I could carry the flaming Harmony Torch while running. But somehow, the magic of the run extinguished these doubts, and I went and returned refreshed.

Upon coming home to Seattle from the run, my excitement flowed over into flipping through photos of the welcome ceremony for the run. It was held at the Seattle Center hosted by then–First Lady of Seattle, Pam Schell. We were seated next to

facing: The glories of spring perk up spa guests to Avanyu Spa, La Posada de Santa Fe.

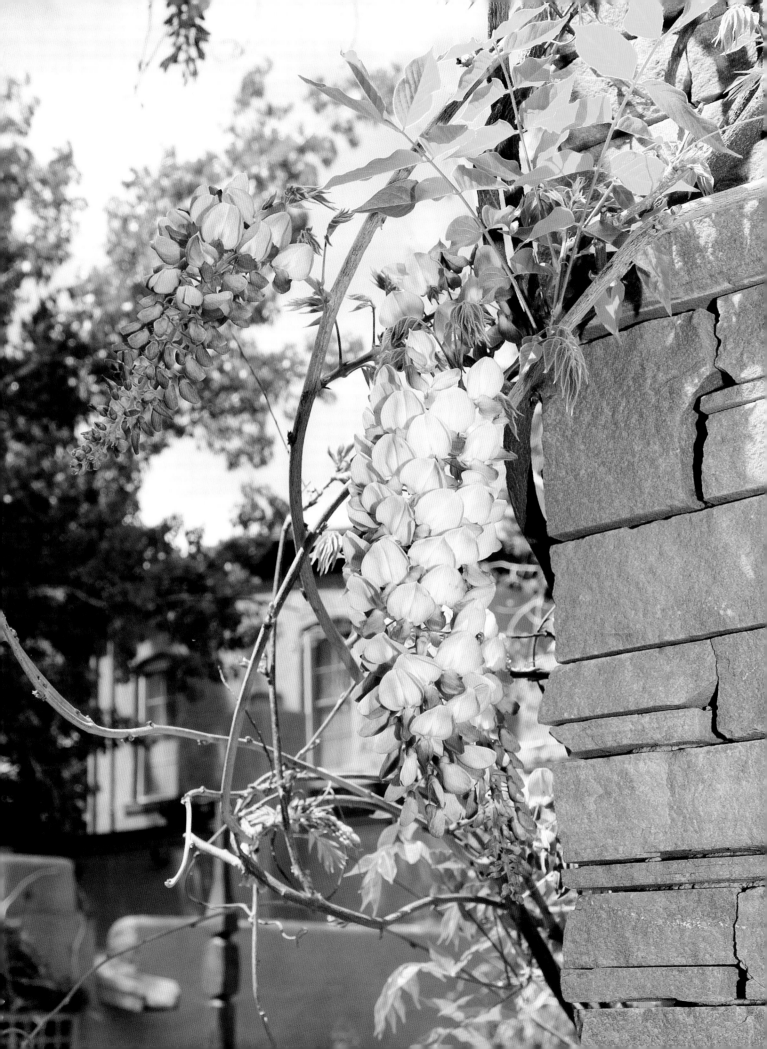

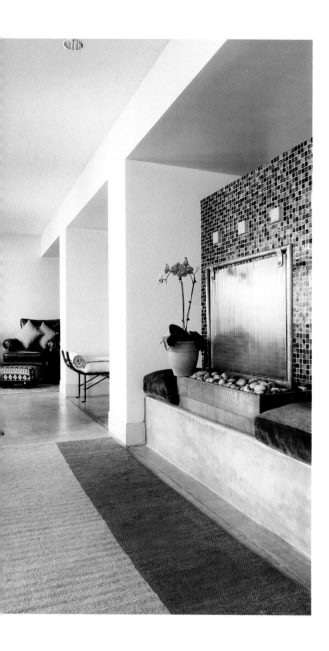

Natural elements of water, stone, and wool carpeting soften the spa waiting room at ShaNah Spa at The Bishop's Lodge north of Santa Fe, New Mexico.

each other on the front row. Then, zoom—photos taken from the back row showed all too clearly, masses of white hair and a thinning spot on the left side of my head. I was horrified and stunned!

This was followed by major dental work including two root canals and crowns, constant fatigue, and an itchy rash on both shins that was a real pain, literally.

After analyzing the food diary of what I ate for a week, my naturopath diagnosed Candida yeast infection. Chipping away at my growing malaise, we worked one step at a time to encourage my body's recovery.

When I started to notice my body changing, I was forty-five. Ten years later, I can honestly look back with gratitude for the experiences my body gave me—in reconnecting with it, and in learning to honor the one and only physical sheath I'm blessed with in this lifetime.

Not only was it literally painful, physically, but emotionally, I was at a loss in acknowledging how much I'd neglected my body, and the helpless feeling of "what to do now?" It was, in a word— depressing. But gradually, as I prayed for help, my daily meditations pulled me back from the brink.

This book is a heartfelt attempt to share what I've learned, to purify and protect *The Body, Humanity's Fort* (and the title of one of Sri Chinmoy's[1] books) from unnecessary harm. Good health is a treasure we prize, but ironically, only after losing it; thank god for learning opportunities while in the process of regaining it too!

Spa Living: Ideas, Tips & Recipes for Revitalizing Body-Mind-Spirit is not a call to indulge in mindless pampering. Rather, it is an effort to recognize the importance of consciously nurturing ourselves to prevent serious physical and emotional imbalances before they happen. An ounce of prevention is truly worth worlds of curative efforts later; it's a new paradigm shift for health-care practitioners and the public to consider, given ever-spiraling health-care costs.

Within the wide parameters constantly being developed in the spa industry, this book focuses on naturally healthful services offered by day and destination spas to promote good health. This book does not cover medical spas.

In the process of discovering self-healing, may you enjoy healing love and delectable bites from nature's organic pharmacy and her biodynamic gardens. It would be inspiring to hear from you too, about your own experiences in embracing nature's exotic spas—from the harvest of your home garden to the local farmers'

[1] Sri Chinmoy, my meditation master since 1980, is founder of the global relay run World Harmony Run, www.worldharmonyrun.org. The focus on this Path for physical and spiritual fitness has always endeared it to me.

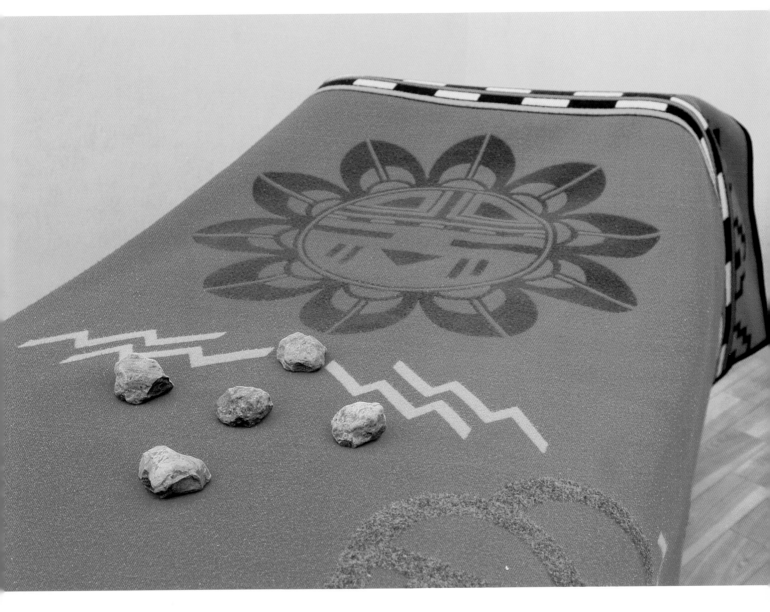

markets you frequent. I can be reached through e-mail at
sunamita@sisna.com.

The final chapter on going green is a subject dear to my
heart. Mother Nature needs our sincere intentions to minimize
pollution in every sense of the word. Let us work together for a
greener, more hopeful world that sustains and benefits everyone.

Detail of a Pendleton wool blanket at
Nidah Spa, Eldorado Hotel, Santa Fe,
New Mexico. The sacred Native American
medicine wheel honors north for restora-
tion, east for renewal, south for vitality,
and west for purification, while the golden
center balances it all.

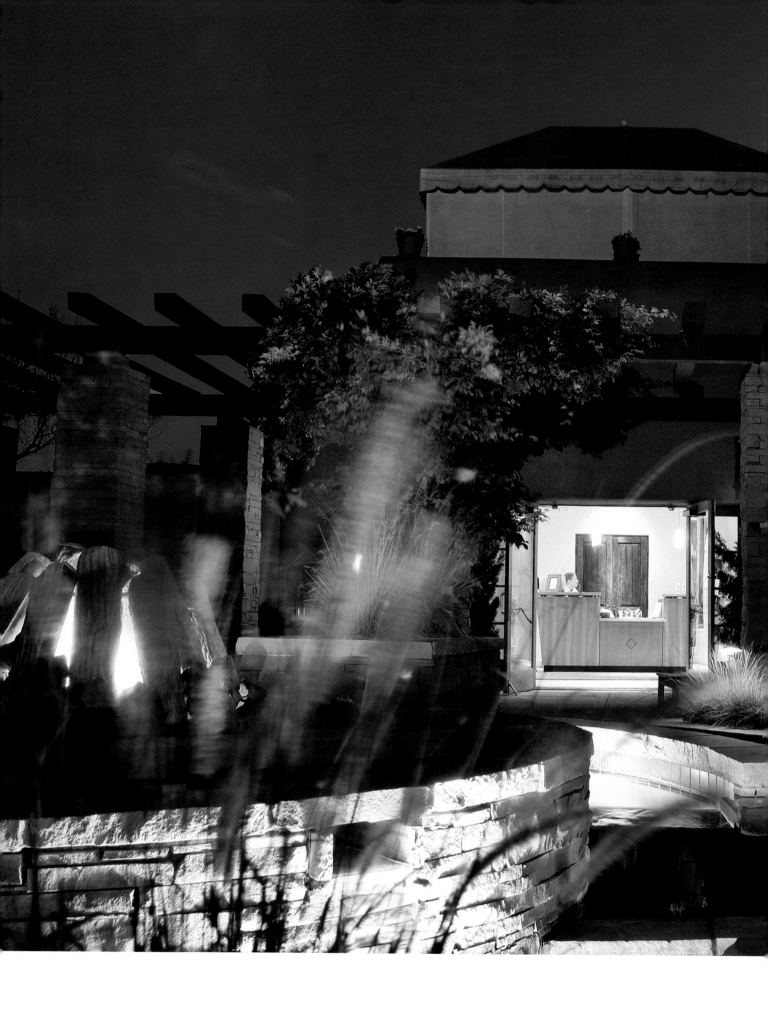

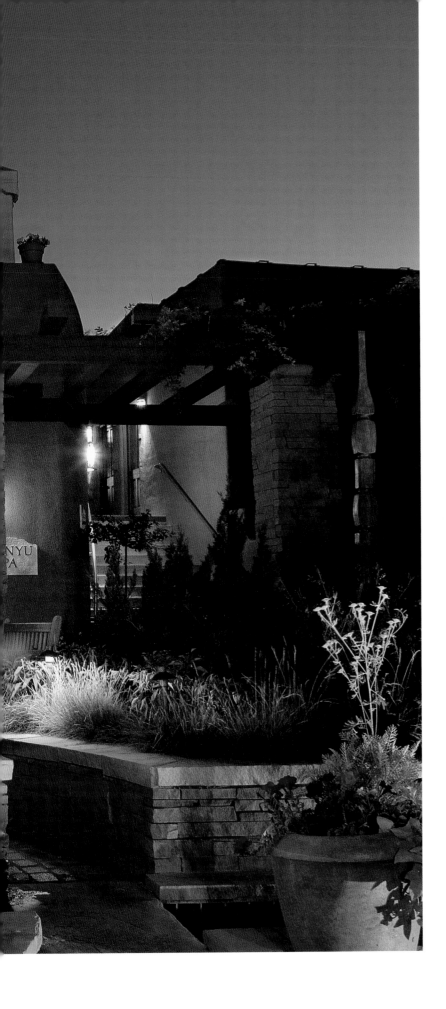

Dusk sets an inviting mood to luxuriate in evening spa sessions at La Posada de Santa Fe Resort & Spa. (Courtesy photo)

CHAPTER ONE

THE QUEST FOR RADIANT BEAUTY AND WELL-BEING

Beauty is from within and expressed on the face.
Beauty does not have a recipe, but is expressed in
how one manages the movement of life.

—Deborah Szekely, founder of "The Original Destination
Fitness Resort & Spa," Rancho La Puerta

The eternal quest for radiant good health continues challenging societies to present outer beauty on center stage, or at the very least, the appearance thereof. Ancient Egyptian civilizations appeared to Greek historian Herodotus to put cleanliness above seemliness in their pursuit of good health. Together with their predilection for cosmetics and beauty care, cleanliness exemplified the importance of good grooming and breeding.

Doubtless, the desire to be clean and pleasant to the olfactory senses was necessitated by desert conditions, exacerbated by the blazing sun and drying winds of Egypt. Thousands of years ago, black kohl eyeliner was used for beauty, protection from the hot sun, and for healing. Today, Egyptian women still use kohl (an Arabic word), as do women in the Middle East and Indian subcontinent.[1]

And just as the ancient Egyptians were adept at working with nature's topographical constraints (as their monuments and landscaping ingenuity testified), they were also highly knowledgeable about nature's pharmacy and utilized herbs, spices, flowers, and plants for healing. For example, perfumes used gum resins such as myrrh, flowers such as lilies and irises, and herbs and spices such as marjoram and cinnamon, in their recipes.[2]

However, much of this information has been resurrected from archeological digs and not much from actual, continuous practice, ancient as it is.

The more recent ancient traditions of beauty and healing that have survived, and are as powerful today, instead come from *Ayurveda*, sacred scientific knowledge from India rooted in over

An amethyst in the steam room at New York's Mandarin Oriental Spa helps refocus scattered energy. (Courtesy photo)

---

[1] Joyce Tyldesley's chapter on "Good Grooming" in *Daughters of Isis: Women of Ancient Egypt* notes both men and women used cosmetics for health and beauty reasons then too.
[2] Lise Manniche, *Sacred Luxuries: Fragrance, Aromatherapy, and Cosmetics in Ancient Egypt.*

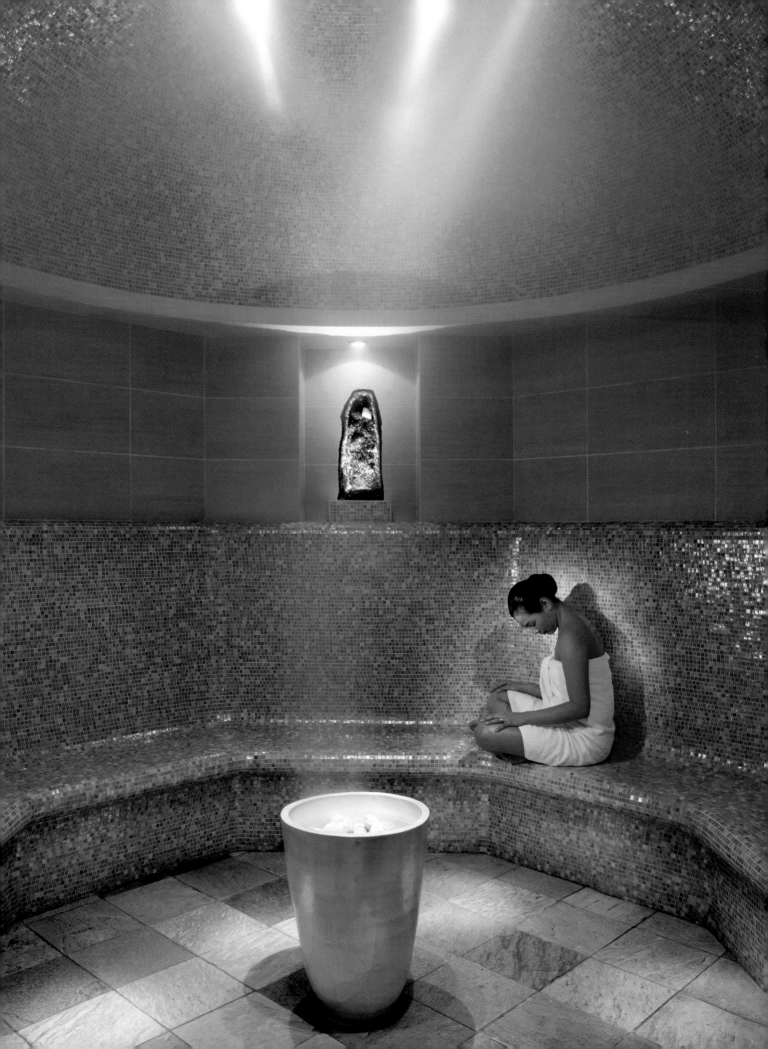

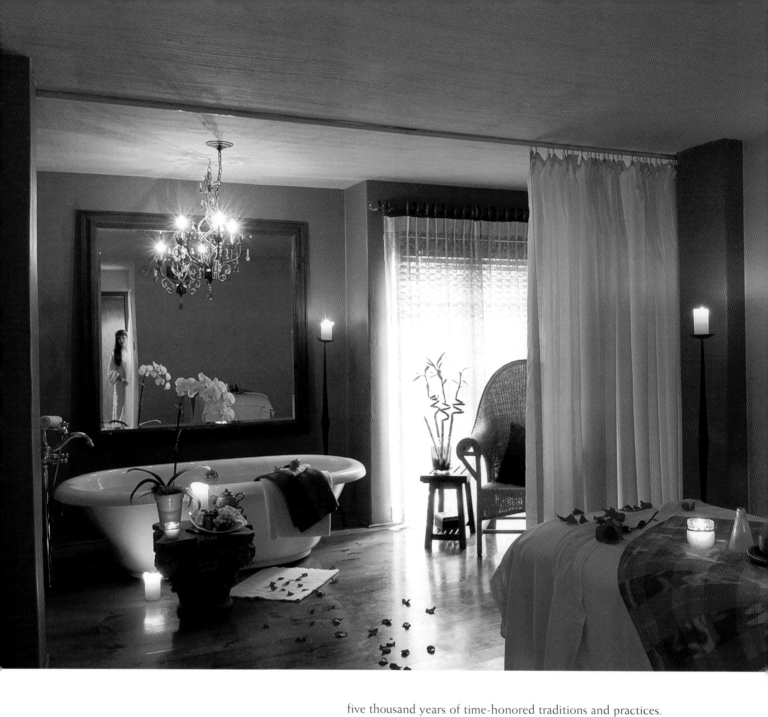

five thousand years of time-honored traditions and practices.

Ayurveda means "the science of life" in Sanskrit, culled from the *Atharva Veda*, the fourth and last of the sacred Hindu texts called the *Rig Veda*. Over the centuries, Ayurveda has influenced many western modalities of healing such as homeopathy, aromatherapy, psychiatry, meditation, nutrition, and polarity therapies. These are among the myriad services now offered by every beauty and health spa in the world, with some ingeniously adapted to local exotic materials and rituals, and whole-heartedly embraced by spa guests who keep returning for more.

"The beauty of Ayurveda is that it recognizes every individual as [having] a unique psycho-physiological makeup, with their own basic constitution from conception on, and therefore promotes

Setting the mood at SpaTerre, Santa Fe, for a leisurely spa-style bath with aromatic candles, fresh flowers, and muted lighting.

customized self-healing, with the assistance of a trained practitioner," says Dr. Ed Danaher, director of the Panchakarma Department at The Ayurvedic Institute in Albuquerque, New Mexico.

More intrinsically, Danaher points out the interrelatedness of body-mind-spirit in promoting overall good health in a person. And although a person new to Ayurveda would need the guidance of a trained practitioner in the beginning, it is a healing process that becomes, ultimately, "self-healing," when the person becomes more skilled with preparations on their own, that are relevant to their own *dosha* or constitutional type.

According to Ayurveda, the three types of dosha—*vata, pitta,* and *kapha*—balance out the person by bestowing a state of natural beauty with good health, happiness, and a sense of well-being. This, then, is the gold standard of Ayurveda—personalized beauty care and eating for radiant health that contributes to a person's intuitive ability for self-healing, to live a more fulfilling life from deep within.

Lest this sounds like a lone voice from Danaher, Donald Kimon Lightner, licensed acupuncturist at Miraval Resort and Spa in Tucson, Arizona, sings a similar refrain too. Miraval is consistently voted a top destination spa by readers of lifestyle and travel magazines such as *Conde Nast Traveler* and *Travel and Leisure*.

"Radiant health and real beauty comes from having a lot of love and compassion, a love of life, and living a beautiful life. We are what we eat, what we think, what decisions we make, and what we value—and these activities are constantly changing. I am always working to clean myself up, to train my mind, and to purify my heart (and find I have a lot of work to do)," Lightner says with a smile.

The goal of Miraval's Whole-Person Healing program is to help the body relax so it can heal. "When the body relaxes, it heals," they say. And this program helps people do just that, with the help of soothing and pain-reducing therapies that it calls "unparalleled." Guests must agree, based on their yearly voting preferences in lifestyle magazines championing Miraval's matchless treatments, many of which are Ayurvedic.[3]

Dr. David Frawley,[4] author of over thirty books on Ayurveda and internationally respected for spreading this science to practitioners outside of India, states, "Ayurveda is a whole new paradigm shift in the science of healing and wellness. Instead of dealing with pathogens [organisms that contribute to disease] and trying to

Poised for a turquoise-inspired treat at Nidah Spa, Eldorado Hotel, Santa Fe, New Mexico.

---

[3] Amy Gunderson reported in the *New York Times* (October 14, 2005) that guests are lining up to buy Miraval's newest spa-related real estate innovation—spa condos with each unit sporting its own meditation space and a private outdoor courtyard.
[4] Frawley is also president of the American Institute of Vedic Studies, whose board members include Dr. Deepak Chopra.

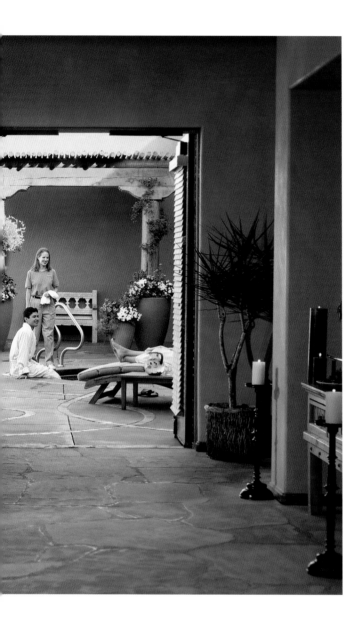

Guests enjoy the outdoor pool at Tamaya Mist Spa & Salon. (Courtesy photo)

facing: An antique tapestry frames one wall of Cal-a-Vie's library. (Courtesy photo)

destroy them with futile attempts, as they are very much part of the eco-system, Ayurveda instead works on strengthening the immune system. Food is paramount, as food makes up the body's cells and tissues. We are what we eat. And, we also need to address lifestyle practices that may drain and weaken a person's vitality." Such draining habits include constantly being on the run, without giving the body time to balance itself with quiet time and downtime.

Unequivocally advocating the beautiful self-healing science that Ayurveda is, through unlocking the life force called *prana* (also called *qi* in Chinese and *mana* in Hawaiian), Frawley emphasizes, "Health begins when you consciously live life on a daily basis. In this country, about 25 percent of young children are already on medication—an extremely high proportion. What's going to happen when they get older? Besides, why keep spending money on expensive medicines with prices continuously spiraling, and putting up with unwelcome side effects that won't go away?" He points out it's a different matter for catastrophic injuries, for which Ayurveda, like western medical practice, also offers medical intervention with surgery.

Instead, Frawley urges, *"make more time"*—for quiet time, time to enjoy a meal, taking time off from work for healing, and setting aside meditation time every day for internal fine tuning. He wryly observes how ironic it is that some who earn high incomes do not have the time to spare in further enriching their body's good health.

In Europe, recognizing the need for downtime to heal and recuperate even resonates in eastern European countries governed by dictators. "When my country was ruled by Nicolae Ceausescu (1918–89), every citizen was given three weeks of free spa treatments every year, in all of Romania's spas," said noted aesthetician Cornelia Zicu, who opened a luxury day resort—the Cornelia Luxury Day Resort—on New York's Fifth Avenue in January 2005, sporting the first *watsu* pool in the city.

Predating Nobel Laureate Linus Pauling's cutting-edge discoveries of *Vitamin C and the Common Cold* (the title of his best-selling book), for which he was awarded the Nobel Prize in 1954, Hungarian Dr. Albert von Szent-Györgyi was awarded the Nobel Prize for Medicine in 1937 for his

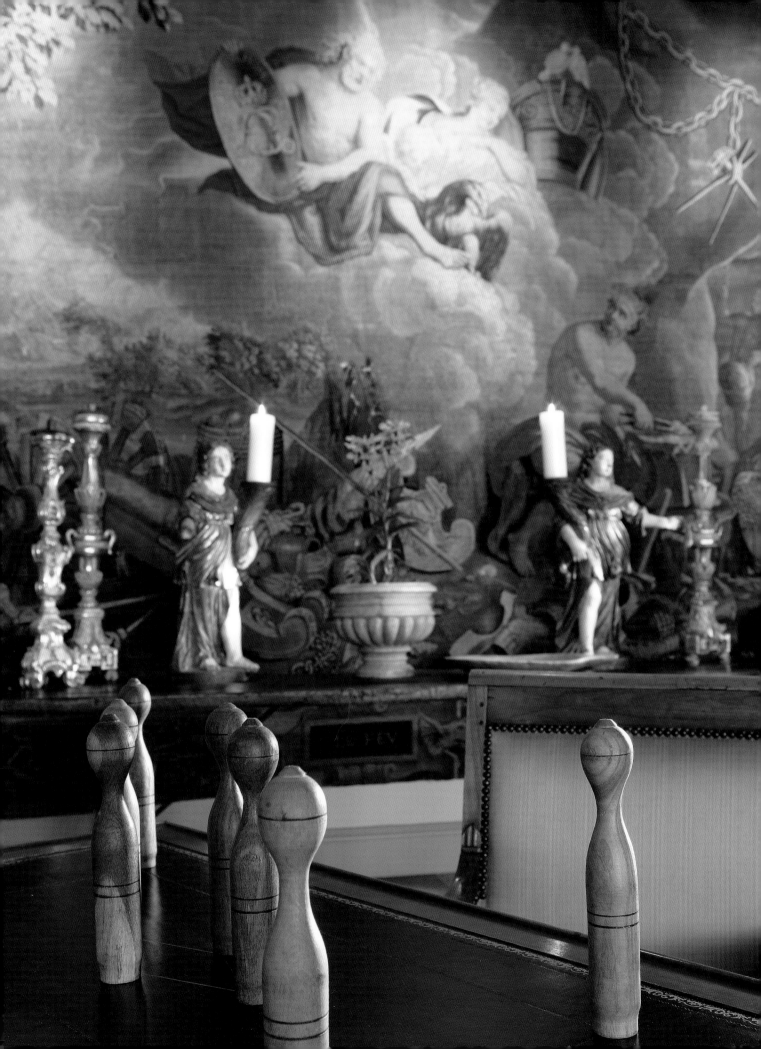

work on identifying vitamin C and cell metabolism.

Szent-Györgyi showed how cells were altered by internal and external stresses that disturbed cellular metabolic rates for regular, healthy oxidation. Ultimately, the immune system was so adversely affected that pathogens took over the distressed cells, and disease set in—until vitamin supplementation and rest rebalanced cellular functions again.

In Ayurveda, the poetic diagnosis for imbalance proclaims a state of "*pragya parad*, where disease begins with a mistake of the intellect," notes Dr. Ed Danaher, "where accumulating habits compound, to worsen the condition, over time."

With his quick wit, Lightner quips, "When there is less thinking, and ideas about things, we can see the universe in its original radiant beauty without adding our silly notions to it. A beautiful person is at ease and in love with life. There is even a Nat King Cole song about this. Such a person is kind and gentle, but disciplined; and ethical and firm with their values, but not belligerent about them. A beautiful person practices generosity and modesty, and appreciates the Simple, Ordinary, Things in Life."

Lightner shares his favorite poem from Zen master Han-shan Te-Ch'ing, who is credited with reviving Buddhism when the Ming dynasty (1368–1644) was crumbling in China:

A hundred thousand words are flowers in the sky

A single body mind is moonlight on the water

When information stops and the cunning ends

At this place there is no place for thought.

—Han-shan Te-Ch'ing (1546–1623)

From all over continental America, including Rancho La Puerta in Tecate, Mexico, the first North American destination spa started by Deborah Szekely and her late husband, Edmond, in 1940, the resounding messages are clear:

26

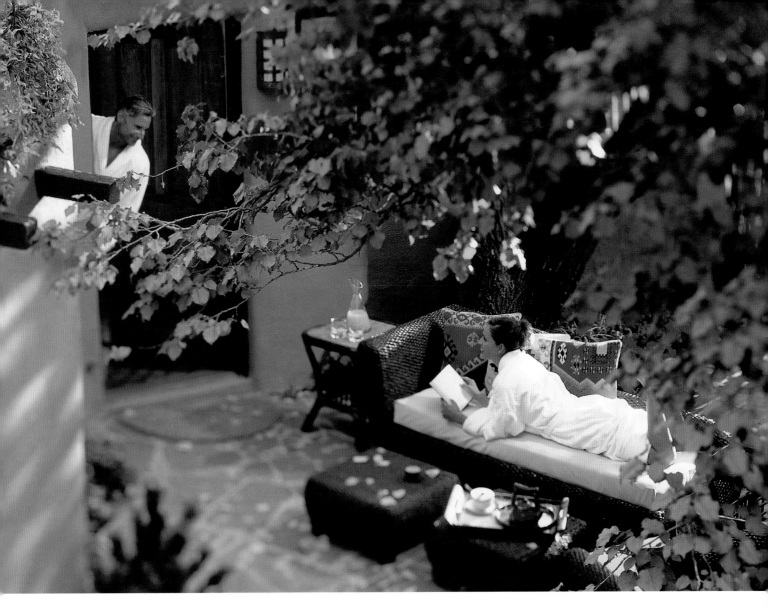

- It is up to the individual to consciously *want* to make positive decisions that impact, and reward, with quality of life that sparkles with vibrant, healing energy;

- To recognize these lifestyle decisions as coming from *within*, in respecting the soul's light that is the foundation (from conscience to the voice of intuition) for all good actions—waiting to be tapped for outer action, guidance, and protection; and

- A person's powerful immune system stems from a *balanced body-mind-spirit* that radiates outer vitality and good health.

The following chapters discuss nature's healing pharmacy with spa treatments that promote natural well-being from within—including facials for women and men, physical fitness, good food for good moods, and meditation. Plus, sensible new "green" ideas to try at home for abundant, holistic health that resonates in humans and with the environment.

Relaxing between spa sessions at La Posada de Santa Fe Resort & Spa. (Courtesy photo)

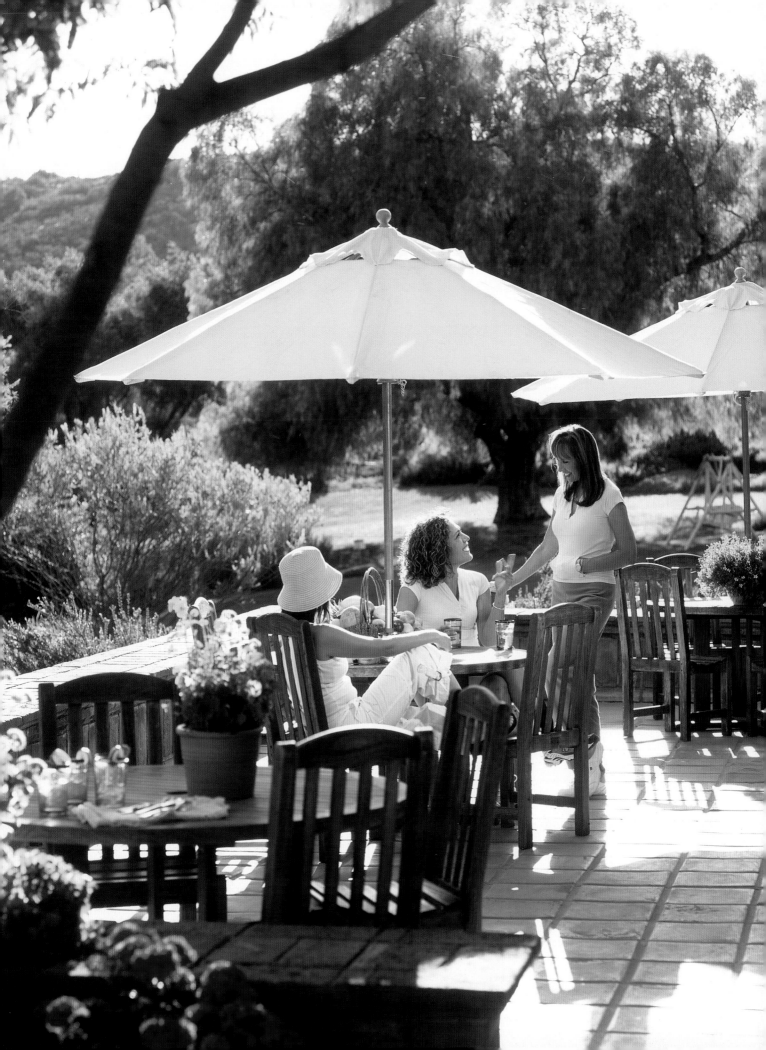

This special section graphically illustrates the chapter's vision with these striking quotes and images, based on answers from different experts to one question:

What makes for a beautiful person and why?

What makes a beautiful person? "Someone who glows from within. This glow is evident when a person is: content, in harmony with the environment, at ease with the situations they are in, and at peace with themselves. Invariably, this is reflected in their body and facial expressions—the way they move, speak, and

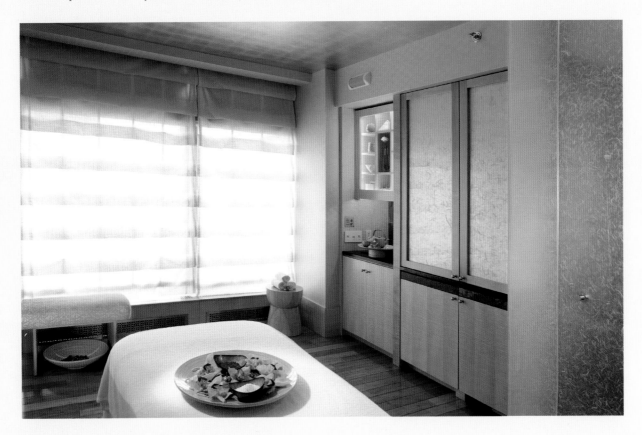

act—which is ultimately their own unique beauty. A balanced person is a good-looking person. By 'balanced,' I mean the physical, mental, emotional, and spiritual aspects of their being. When they are fulfilled by these elements, they are content, and reflect true inner beauty." —*Kiki Osada, Operations Manager, Mandarin Oriental Spa, New York, New York*

"[A beautiful person does] the best with what she has, and is very happy with the reflection that looks back at her. This individual feels

facing: Spa guests become "patio pals" at Rancho la Puerta. (Courtesy photo)

A neutral palette helps spa guests relax at New York's Mandarin Oriental Spa. (Courtesy photo)

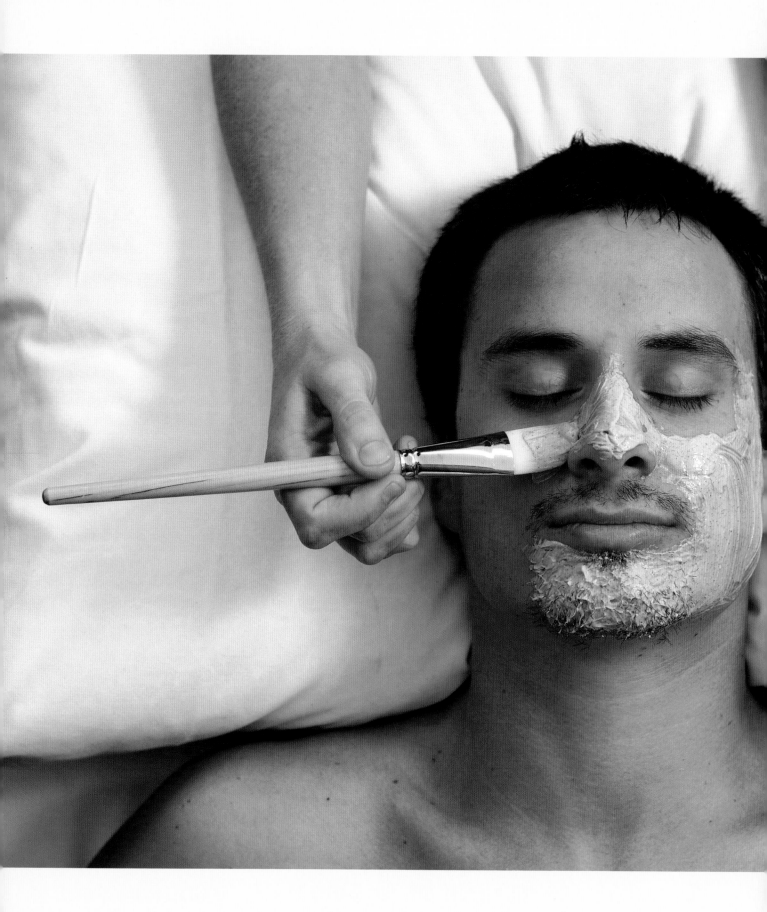

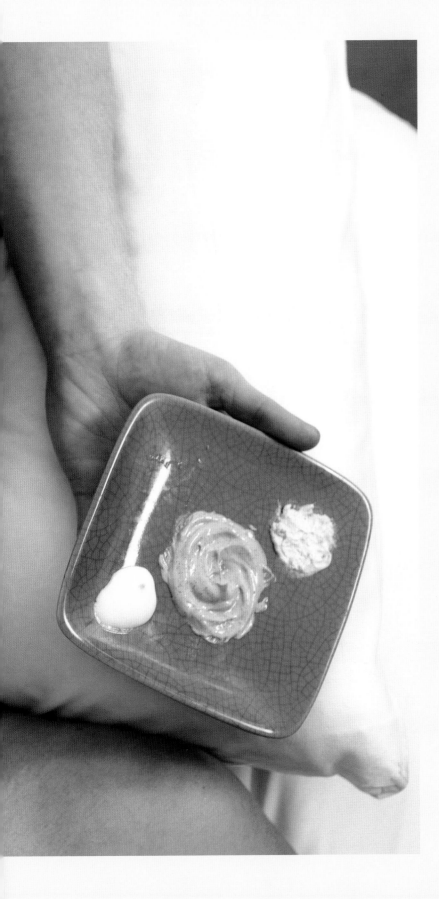

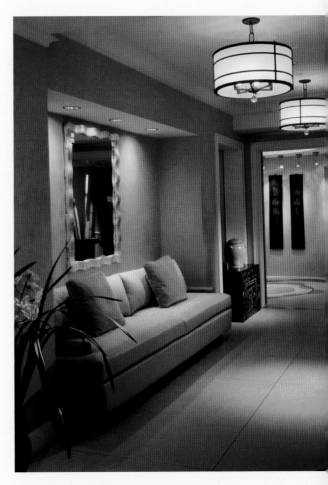

"[A beautiful person does] the best with what she has, and is very happy with the reflection that looks back at her."

left: Regular facials and skin exfoliation for men minimize ingrown facial hair. (Courtesy, Tamaya Mist Spa & Salon)

A quiet alcove inspired by the orient invites a pause at Nob Hill Spa at The Huntington Hotel in San Francisco. (Courtesy photo)

"A lovely person . . . take[s] good care of themselves, and their friends and family."

beautiful from the inside out, and it shows by the way she carries herself—meaning her posture and gait, and the way she dresses with dignity and confidence. Something about her demands attention—whether it's her eyes, hair, clothing, posture, or smile." —*Jan Greaves, Director of Skin Care, Rancho La Puerta Fitness Resort and Spa, Tecate, Mexico*

"A lovely person is well-grounded inwardly and spiritually. Their thoughts and their words speak to gracious actions that nurture themselves and others positively." —*James Leemon, Psychologist and Owner, Terme di Aroma Spa, Philadelphia, Pennsylvania*

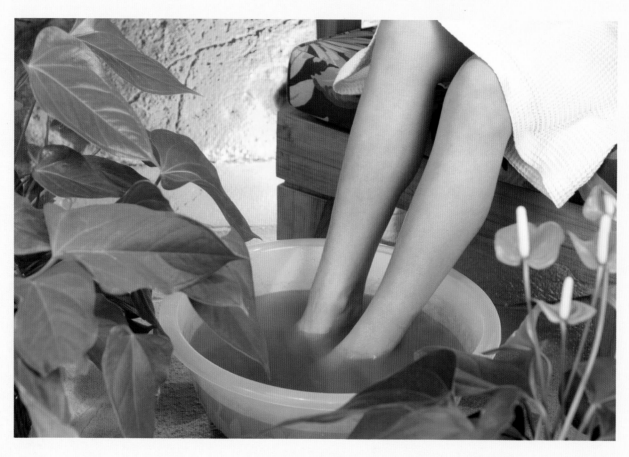

"A lovely person is happy, centered, full of good energy, and embraces the spirit of aloha or sincere love in their hearts for humanity. They take good care of themselves, and their friends and family." —*Gary Rohana, Director, SpaOlakino, Honolulu, Hawaii*

"Looking beautiful comes from within. When you take good care of yourself (with proper diet, exercise, and a good skin-care regimen including sun protection), you feel good about that internally, and it will show on the outside too. Take pride in *who* you are, and allow it to reflect on *how* you put yourself together each day. This will create a domino effect—you will look sharp, confident, and beautiful." —*Andrea Miller, Manager, Golden Door Skin Care at Golden Door, Escondido, California*

"Beauty is not simply skin deep. Beauty encompasses all aspects of a person—mind, body, and soul—with each aspect key to achieving ultimate beauty. It's quite amazing! When a person is of sound mind, body, and spirit, they have a very distinct glow." —*Hippo Lipkin, Spa Director, Mandara Spa Hawaii, LLC, Hilton Hawaiian Village, Honolulu, Hawaii*

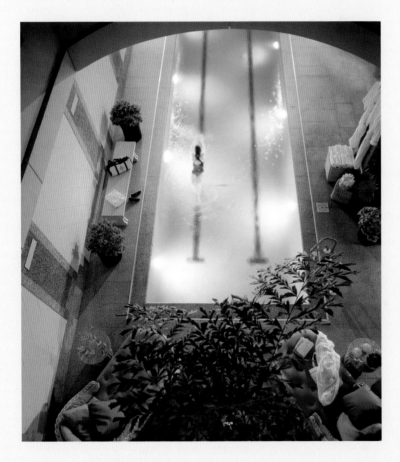

"An attractive person has healthy, glowing skin, hair, nails, and teeth; weight proportioned to body frame; a current style of dress that's not necessarily trendy; and natural-looking make up." —*Jenean La Roche, Director, Nob Hill Spa, San Francisco, California*

"Beauty in a person comes from within. There are some people who are extremely grounded and confident from within, radiating an amazing energy that you cannot help but notice—and say, 'how

"Take pride in who you are, and allow it to reflect on how you put yourself together each day."

facing: Soaking in Epsom salts is an easy way to bring relief to sore feet at the end of the day. (Courtesy of SpaOlakino)

A quick dip in the pool refreshes immediately.

33

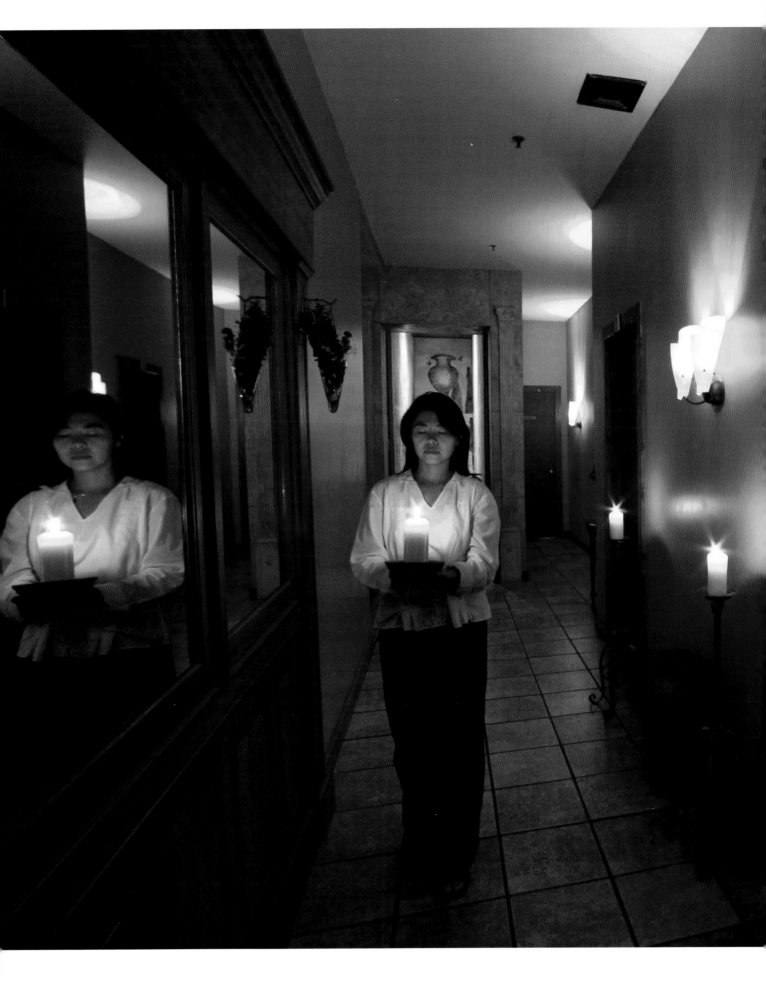

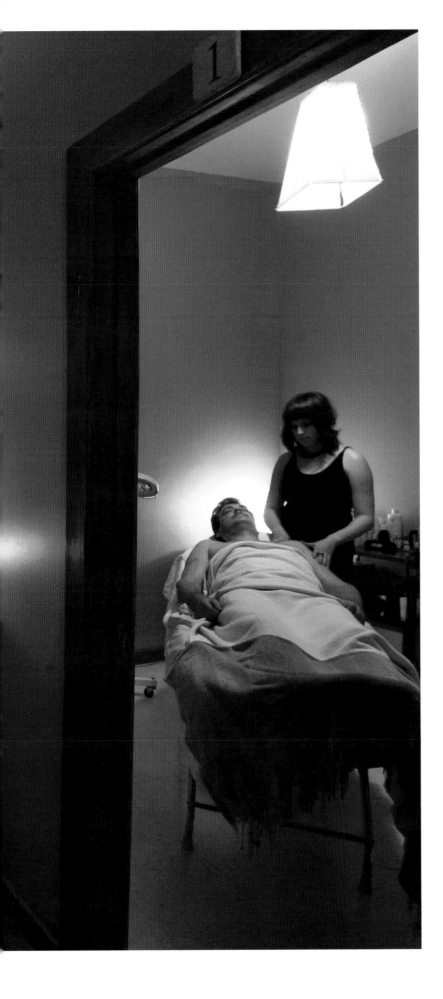

Terme di Aroma's exotic surroundings in the heart of Philadelphia. (Courtesy photo)

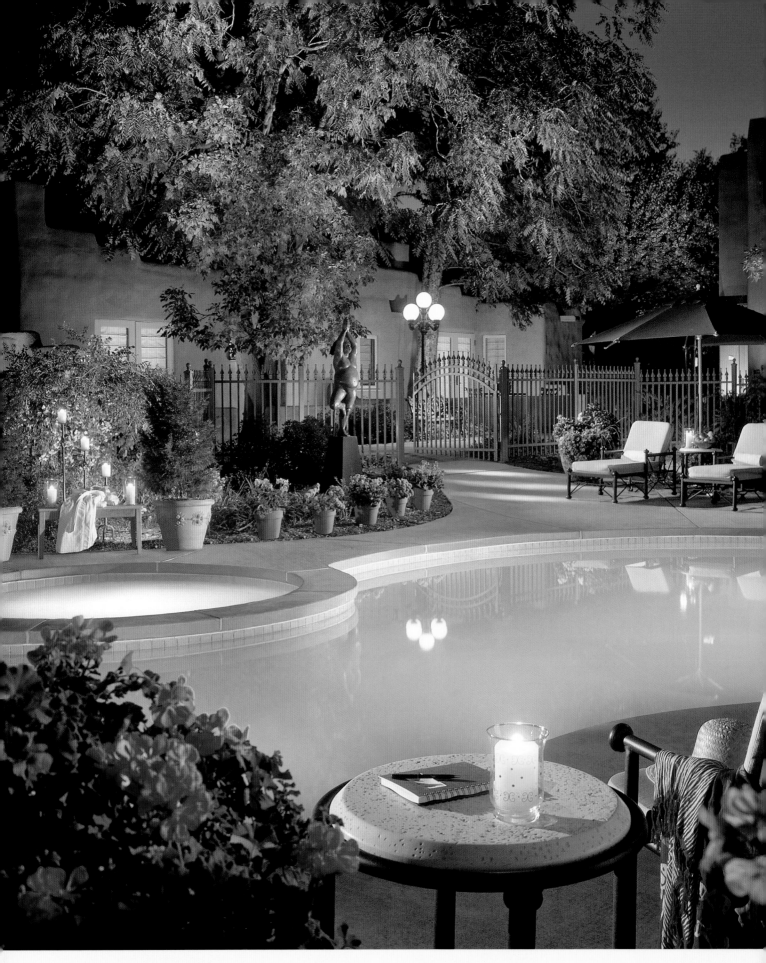

Unwinding by the pool with journaling. (Courtesy,
La Posada de Santa Fe Resort & Spa)

lovely he or she is!'" —*Nicole Morris, Spa Director, The Westin at Times Square, New York, New York*

"What makes someone beautiful is what, and who, they are on the inside. As clichéd as it sounds, if you have strong morals, beliefs, and a sense of who you truly are, and your mission in life is positive, I believe that makes you beautiful!" —*Kim Telles, Spa Manager, Tamaya Mist Spa & Salon, Hyatt Regency Tamaya Resort & Spa, Santa Ana Pueblo (north of Albuquerque), New Mexico*

"To me, beauty starts on the inside and works its way out."

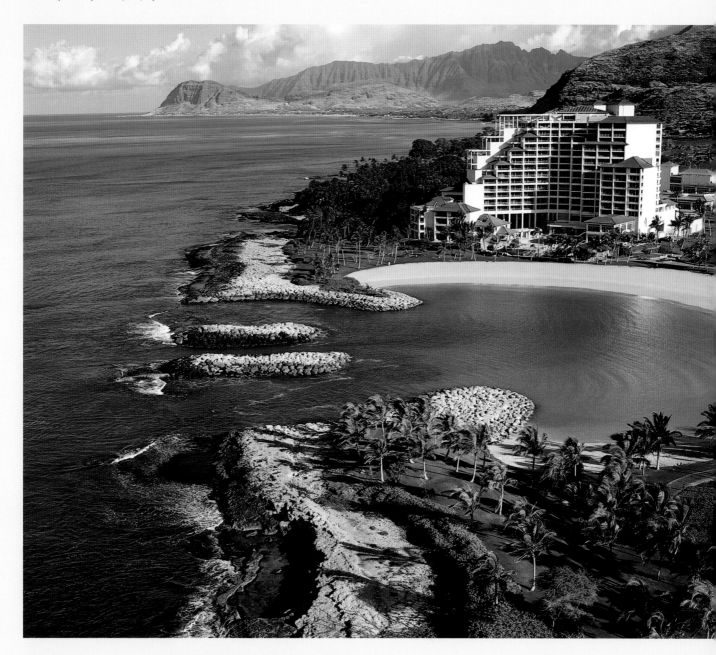

The natural gem-like setting of Ihilani Resort and Spa on Oa'hu Island in Hawaii encourages natural healing. (Courtesy photo)

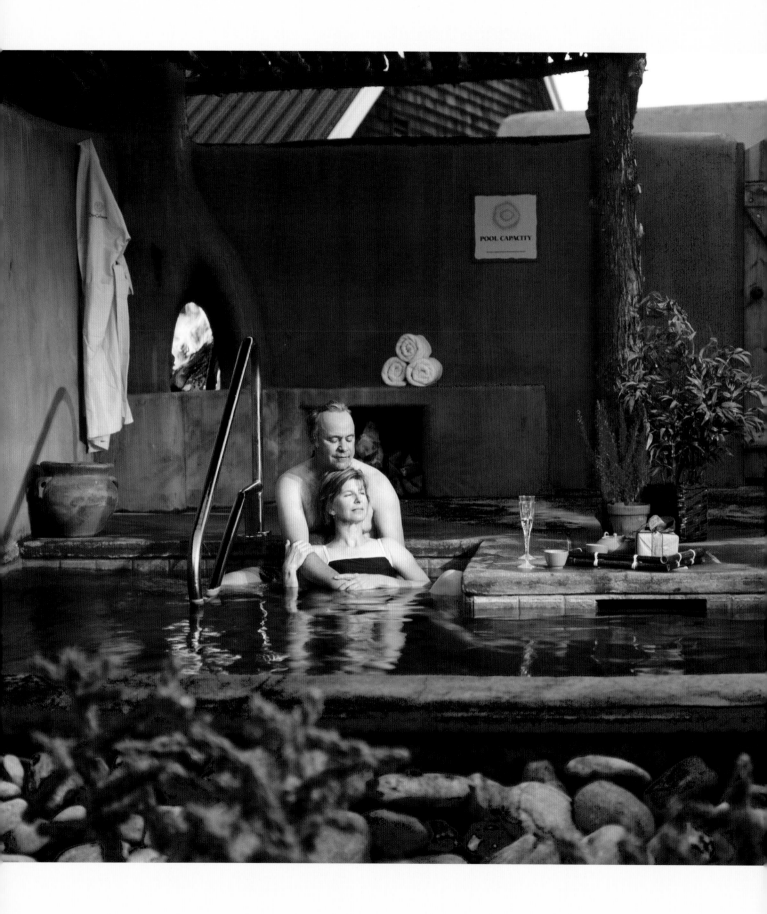

"The inner beauty counts above all else. We see this in the person's attitude, sparkling eyes, and most of all, their happy smiles."
—*Suk Mancinelli, Manager, Four Seasons Spa, New York*

"While growing up in Romania, I remember how beautiful my grandmother's hands were—soft, smooth, and so young-looking, like a five-year-old's. She loved gardening and cooking. She would scoop out pumpkin with her bare hands and bake it for dessert. The plant enzymes that her hands came into constant contact with nourished her skin immensely." —*Cornelia Zicu, Owner, Cornelia Luxury Day Resort, New York, New York*

"To me, beauty starts on the inside and works its way out. This means doing things that make you feel good about yourself. Eating healthy foods, regular exercise, good hydration of the entire body, a proper balance between work and play—all contribute to inner and outer beauty. Skin becomes healthier, you feel better about your body (even if you're carrying a few extra

"Taking care of your skin and body not only makes you look good, but also makes you feel good, and look radiant."

facing: **Relaxing in a private pool at Ojo Caliente. (Courtesy photo)**

A neutral palette softens a treatment room at Cornelia Day Resort & Spa. (Courtesy photo)

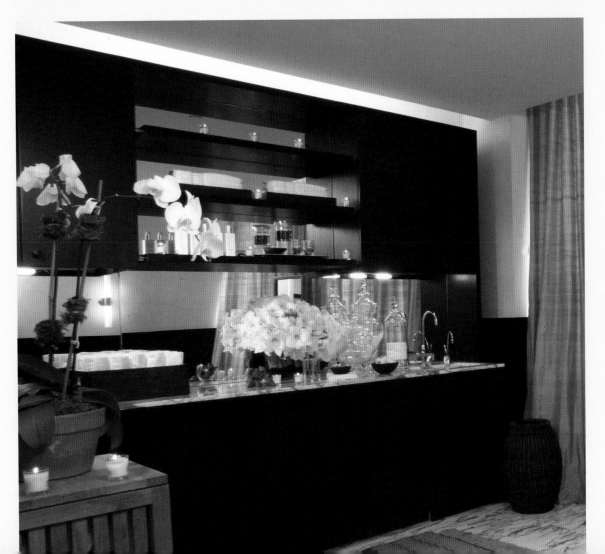

"The inner beauty counts above all else."

pounds), you smile more, and people recognize this and respond accordingly." —*Dan Mohr, Avanyu Spa Director, La Posada de Santa Fe, New Mexico*

"Taking care of your skin and body not only makes you look good, but also makes you feel good, and look radiant. You carry that internal and external glow that is very obvious to everyone around you. Guests are slowly but surely starting to understand the meaning of 'Holistic' treatments versus 'Cosmetic' treatments. As a holistic spa, we educate guests about the difference between the two—that you still get the same results in a more natural way with holistic treatments. More men are coming for facials too. The holistic facial has a lot more massage components to it than a cosmetic facial. Ultimately, you feel as relaxed as you would after a body massage." —*Penny Kriel, Spa Director, Mandarin Oriental Hotel, Washington, D.C.*

Floating away with a facial at The Westin at Times Square. (Courtesy photo)

facing: The Four Seasons Hotel and Spa in Philadelphia sheds tropical ambiance at poolside. (Photography by Ruth Hirshey)

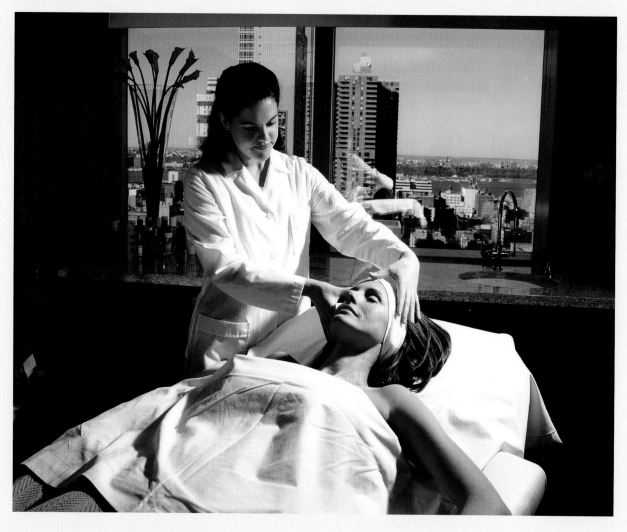

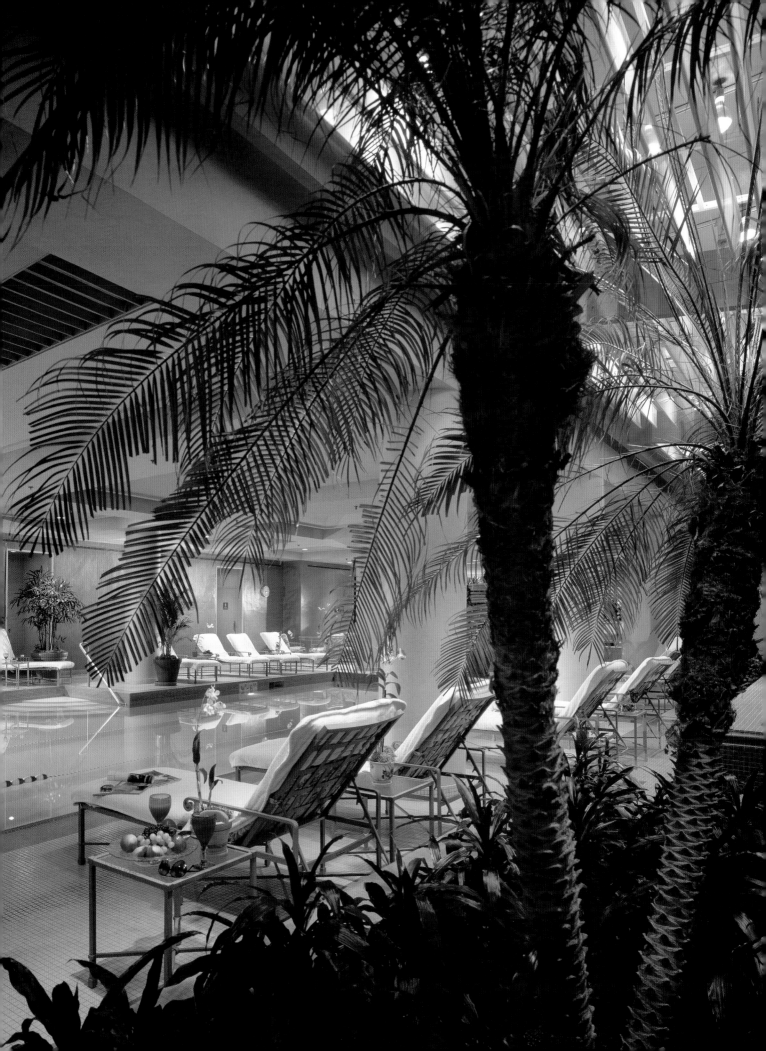

CHAPTER TWO

AN INTRODUCTION TO SPAS AND SERVICES

On a personal level, Cal-a-Vie is the perfect place to go and reenergize from the hectic schedule of a busy life. I have been many times and each time, enjoy it more. It is beautiful in every way—landscape, décor, and facilities. It is small, and so very peaceful. The staff-guest ratio (4-1) is abundant, and gracious with their services.

—Cynthia Harriss, President, GAP North America

The explanation that Cynthia Harriss gives for frequenting a destination spa such as Cal-a-Vie to reenergize from a hectic professional life is the most common reason spa aficionados give for returning. With her myriad responsibilities as president of a mega clothing empire (GAP, North America), the spa's convenient location just north of San Diego, California, facilitates quick getaways for this guest from San Francisco.

And as day and night rhythmically weave with nature's daily tempo, so too the necessity for everyone to rebalance the cadence of living a full, dynamic life—with the need to refill on moments of serenity and inner reflection to promote mental clarity and to stabilize emotions. It's not only emotional energies that need refreshing, but for body cells to also benefit from the opportunity to pause, detoxify, and rejuvenate again.

In other words, taking time out for spa treatments is a health prevention measure that can alleviate major medical problems down the line—well worth their expense, and with the added advantage of enjoying these sessions—as opposed to expending even more resources lying in bed in a sterile hospital room, after medical symptoms and pathogenesis have set in.

In Japan, shiatsu is a form of massage that reduces aches, pains, and stress. Yoshio Nakano of Tucson, Arizona, a nationally recognized shiatsu expert, observes, "Health care in the East is not fooled by symptoms after they have manifested. Instead, we are

facing: The waiting room at Cal-a-Vie's Bath House quietly puts guests at ease while awaiting spa treats. (Courtesy photo)

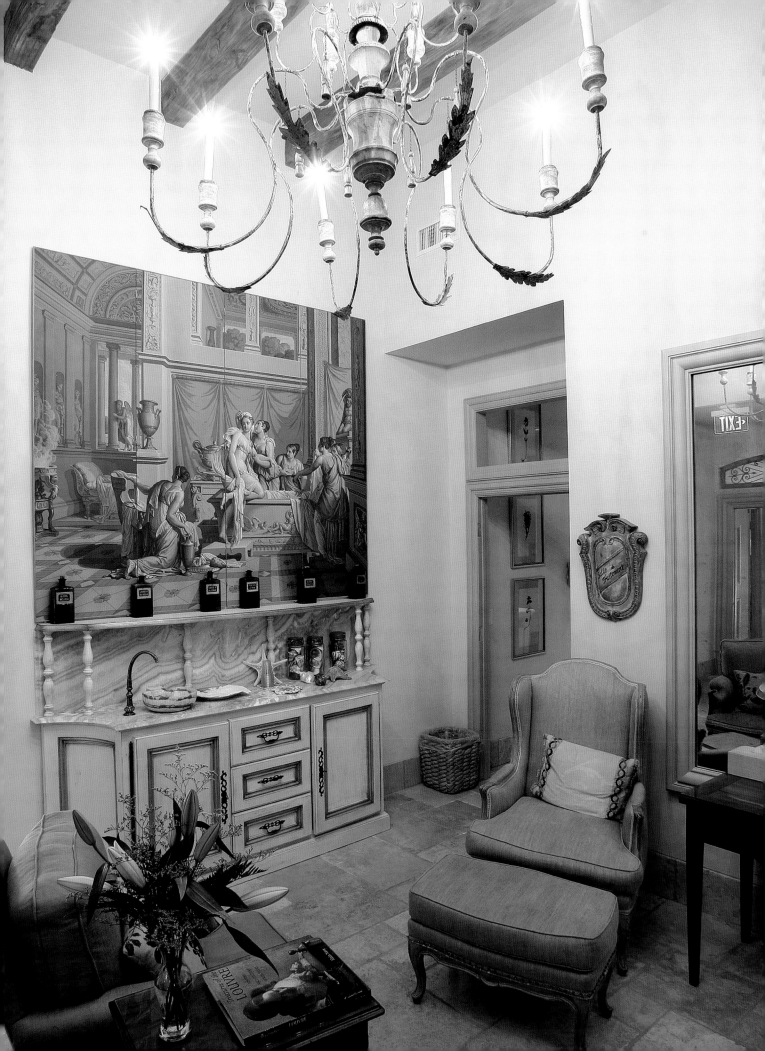

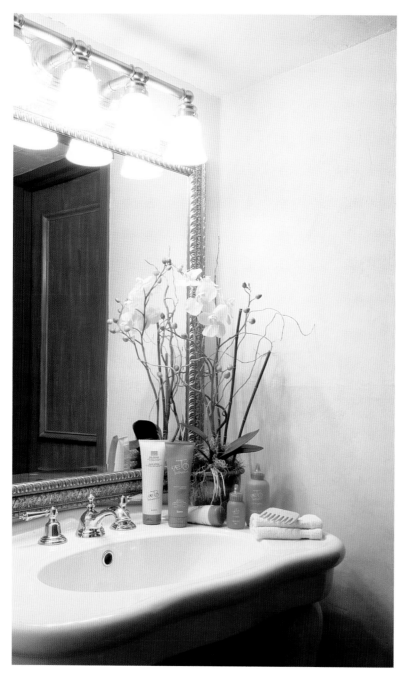

taught to honor the body, be sensitive to its daily needs, and to attend to these needs as they arise." To this end, the Japanese family bathing together in the evening is an exercise in harmony that nurtures family ties and emotional well-being, Nakano points out.

Spa treatments introduce novel explorations of body, mind, and spirit; variations are worked in to complement seasonal changes. Returning guests have a better idea to follow up on treatments that appeal to them, as well as carry out these treatments upon returning home. Invariably, spa experiences turn out to be life-changing epiphanies that enhance daily living, as the examples in these pages show. The benefits for one person can have an impact on other family members, for example, with more nutritious food selection, cooking methods, and exercise. The emotional and psychological rewards are tangible, too, as a person's decidedly positive, upbeat outlook will affect everyone else around them.

"I know I would not be conscious of these exercise needs if it wasn't for Rancho La Puerta," says Sandy Novak of Seattle, who looks forward to her yearly visits to this destination spa in Tecate, Mexico, for benchmark evaluations of how fit she is.[1] Living an active life that improves on, and maintains, quality of life is a strong motivation for Novak to continue exercising and to be at peace with herself and her family.

Joan Messenger's first-person account of her seven-day stay at Cal-a-Vie is a stunning one (see sidebar, page 67). She lost four and a half inches (one and a half inches off her waist, one inch off her hips, one-half inch off each thigh, and one inch off her chest,

Ingredients for a beauty facial scrub in the bathroom.

[1] See chapter 5, Attaining Physical and Emotional Fitness, for Novak's account of her spa experiences, which reflects fitness reasons many returning spa guests give.

SPA TIPS FOR ENJOYING YOUR TREATS(MENTS)

Spa tips from Gloria Ah Sam, SpaHalekulani Director in Honolulu, whose resounding philosophy is "Stay balanced!"

✓ Do not shave for at least four to twelve hours prior to salt or exfoliating services.

✓ Avoid excessive amounts of alcohol consumption for at least twelve hours prior to a spa service.

✓ Don't be afraid to ask questions or ask how to maneuver around the spa facility.

✓ Inform your therapists of any concerns, allergies, or other health issues before your service begins.

✓ Make it clear to your therapists what your expectations are, that is, areas that need attention, sensitivities, results you are trying to achieve, and so forth.

✓ During your treatment, communicate with your therapists about massage pressure, room temperature, in-room music selection or none, excessive skin irritation, or anything that relates to your specific comfort zone and levels.

✓ After your treatment, feel free to discuss issues related to your service, product, or future treatment recommendations.

✓ Remember to drink plenty of water after a treatment involving massage, as toxins are released during the massage process, in addition to the increase of circulation.

✓ If possible, avoid showering off nourishing oils, lotions, or skin treatment products immediately after a body or facial treatment; this will allow your body to absorb them properly.

Note: SpaHalekulani has one of the nicest day spa exit strategies. The guest is invited to assimilate the treatment before leaving, by lounging on the lanai, or patio. Fresh fruit kabobs skewered on coconut sticks and hot hibiscus tea are served. Spa attendants weave in and out of the lanai and your personal space quietly—draping extra towels, if needed, when the wind picks up—solicitous in memorable and kindly ways.

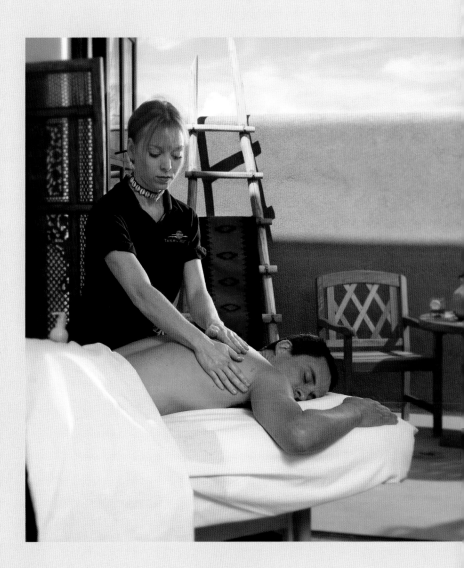

A refreshing massage tones up body muscles.
(Courtesy, Tamaya Mist Spa & Salon)

HOW AROMATHERAPY AND GOOD MEMORIES RELAX AND REVIVE

"Aromatherapy is one of the best ways to stimulate the memory of your Hawaii experience. Fragrances such as plumeria, pikaki, gardenia, and ginger will return you to a renewed sense of island relaxation. Consider also a variety of body and skin-care products, candles, antioxidant supplements, aroma diffusers, and soaps that contain many Hawaiian-inspired healing ingredients such as noni, kukui nut, maile, papaya, coconut milk, awapui, and aloe vera."

—Gloria Ah Sam, Director, SpaHalekulani, Honolulu, Hawaii

Note: The tropical essences of Hawaii can be substituted with the aromas and flavors of other memorable trips you've taken. After returning from a singular trip, I set out trip mementos on a tabletop space, as in an ode or shrine to uncommon experiences. Whenever I need new energy, I pause, give thanks, and recall these memories, which revive with their seemingly never-ending magic.

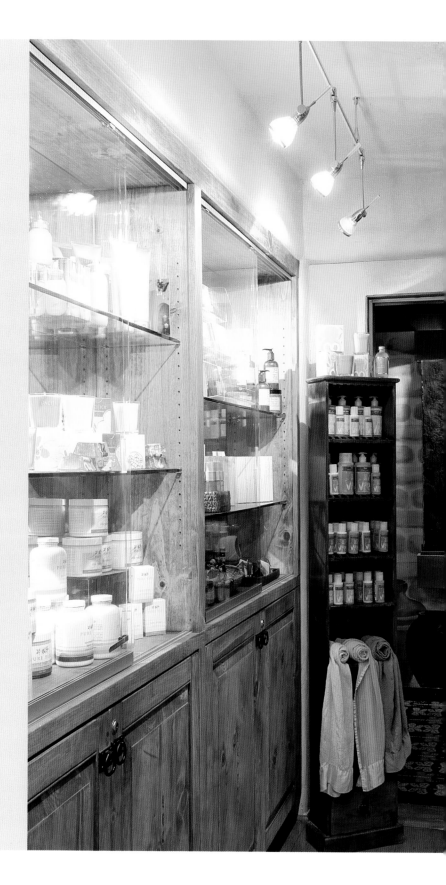

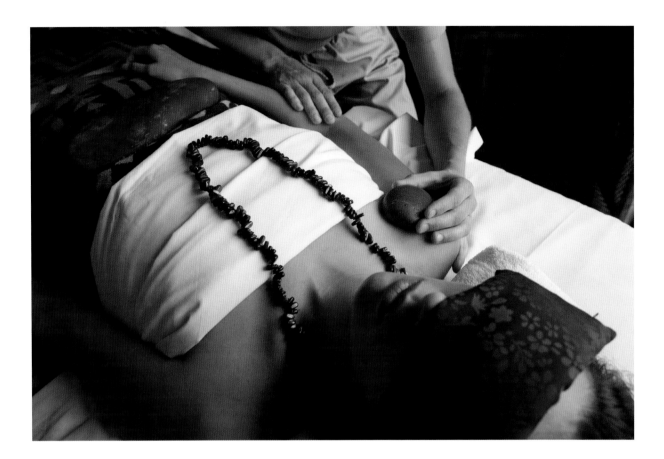

which was primarily back fat) in just seven days.

The payoff? Messenger is now down one dress size and her jeans are two sizes smaller; plus the joie de vivre of hiking and traveling with her husband, six kids, grandchildren, and their dogs. Messenger's remarkable turnaround came about because of two indelible lessons from her spa week—regular exercise to keep off excess calories, and integrating new ways of healthy eating, as she recounts in her story.

Another case of striking *aha!* is from yours truly—when a flash imploded from within to improve my body's immunity. Up till then, six years of living in the high-mountain desert at elevations of over 7,000 feet—while facing extremes of temperatures over a thirty-degree spread every day—had made me think it was the solar intensity, depleted ozone layer, and whipping winds that caused my skin to burn, notwithstanding my use of organic sunscreen lotions laced with UVA and UVB protection.

But after attending various fitness, health, and nutrition sessions fielded by top professionals at Cal-a-Vie and Rancho La Puerta, my soul stirred my mind and body to unlearn old notions

facing: An array of beauty products and a gently falling wall waterfall greet spa guests at the entrance to SpaTerre at The Inn at Loretto in Santa Fe, New Mexico.

Hot stone massage is a popular energizing therapy in spas. (Courtesy, Tamaya Mist Spa & Salon)

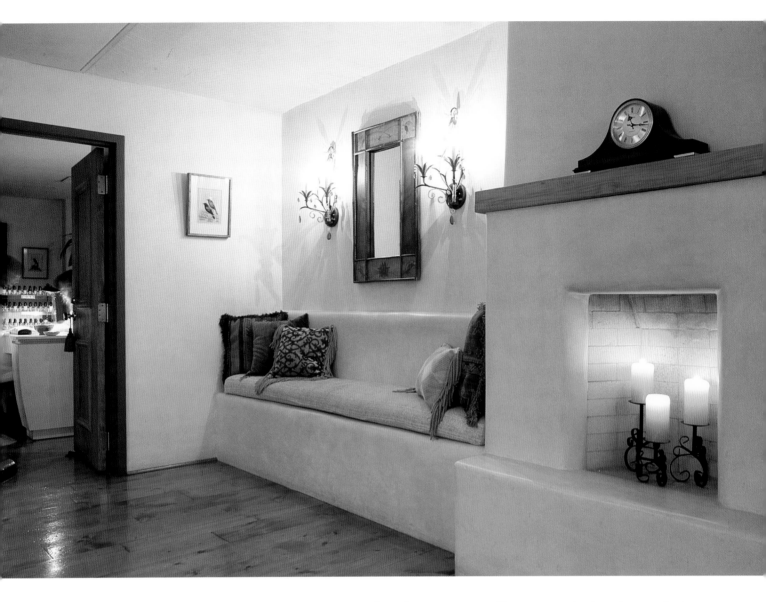

Different kinds of lighting, from candles to wall sconces, echo a warm mood at SpaTerre at The Inn at Loretto in Santa Fe, New Mexico.

in order to learn new ways of honoring my body and caring for it properly. I learned to tune up my immune system.

Destination spas are, undeniably, enjoyable lifestyle retreats. Similar to spiritual retreats, destination spas nurture participants and encourage them to bring out their best, without competing with others, while challenging them to become the very best they can be. Besides being away from it all, gainfully immersed in exciting new life lessons and lifestyle experiences, participants also are able to reattune the senses and be liberated from old ways of thinking and acting. (Read Joan Messenger's engaging account of how she broke the ice with another spa guest on page 68.)

This brings up an important point of keeping an open mind

to allow heartfelt stirrings or intuitive feelings to surface, thus allowing the heart the freedom to resonate and amplify powerful messages from within. This is especially true when tackling new projects on uncertain terrain, as it was for me, when I was at Cal-a-Vie and Rancho La Puerta.

Upon returning, I was motivated to interview even more assiduously, beauty and skin-care experts from across the country on how anyone could enhance their health and immunity, in as many ways as possible. The results are organized into the next three chapters:

• *Incorporating Proper Skin Care*
emphasizes selecting herbal-based items suited to a person's skin type, as the skin mirrors internal health—and an exciting "new" way of tuning in to dosha or constitutional energies that India's Ayurveda practitioners have been harnessing for over five thousand years.

• *Balancing Body-Mind-Spirit with Meditation*
seeks to bring clarity of mind and purpose to all our activities, as well as tapping into deeper levels of spirituality for more meaningful guidance from within.

• *Attaining Physical and Emotional Fitness*
focuses on how important it is to stay emotionally and physically fit by transforming various kinds of energy with our good intentions—from exercise to cooking and eating with a good consciousness—to benefit everyone.

The bottom line: every individual is unique, with very specific health needs. For example, no one product or one product line alone will be the panacea for a person's skin care. Experienced aestheticians will mix and match products from different brands to customize to their client's special needs depending on such factors as the season, travel to a different climate, and events that have stressed out the body and skin.

Tatiana Boncompagni reported in the *Wall Street Journal* (May 12, 2006) The NPD Group's[2] data of "a growing market for high-end facial skin-care creams and lotions, which expanded to $40 million in 2005 from $10 million in 2002." A four-fold sales increase in three years speaks volumes to consumer demands;

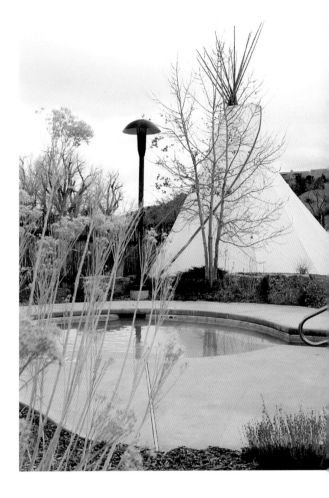

ShaNah Spa at The Bishop's Lodge north of Santa Fe, New Mexico, offers Native American fusions of spa treatments.

[2] Since 1967, The NPD Group, www.npd.com, has been a respected marketing research firm identifying business, technological, and lifestyle trends. NPD is located on Long Island, New York.

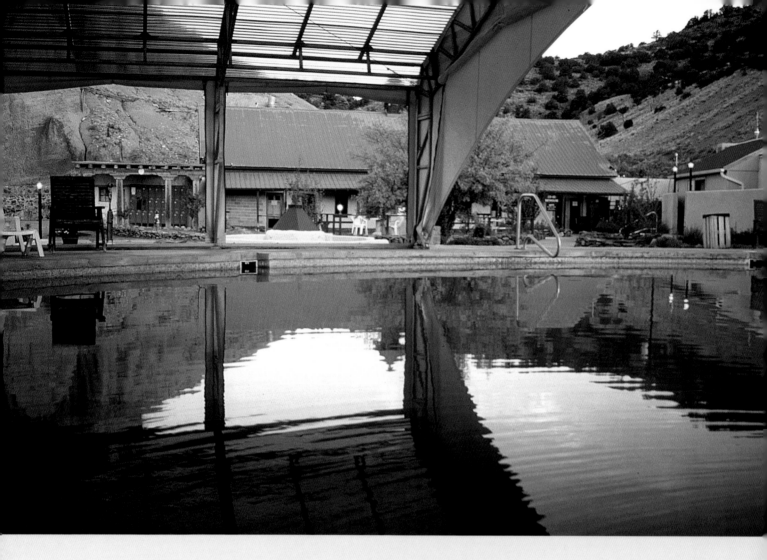

TAKING THE MINERAL WATERS

In Japan and the Mediterranean countries, "taking the waters" is an enjoyable, healthy activity for the entire family.[6] On a larger scale, Japanese families revel in end-of-year excursions to the *onsen*, or mineral springs, for a symbolic purification ritual, to welcome in good luck for the New Year. But the lure of taking to healthful waters is a year-round one everywhere.

In New Mexico, Ojo Caliente is the only mineral springs in the world bubbling up four different mineral waters since time immemorial. If you visit Ojo Caliente, be sure to drink the waters, as well. A brochure describes their curative effects:

- Lithia Spring waters are believed to relieve depression and aid in digestion.
- Iron Spring waters at approximately 109 degrees Fahrenheit are beneficial to the blood and immune system.
- Soda Spring waters aid digestion while relieving digestive problems.
- Arsenic Spring waters at about 103 degrees Fahrenheit relieve arthritis, stomach ulcers, and skin disorders—thereby dispelling notions of Agatha Christie-esque consequences.

Additionally, a mud pool at Ojo Caliente bubbles up clay that, upon slathering on skin, sucks up toxins from the skin as it dries.

---

[6] See accounts in chapter 6, Enjoying Spa Cuisine.

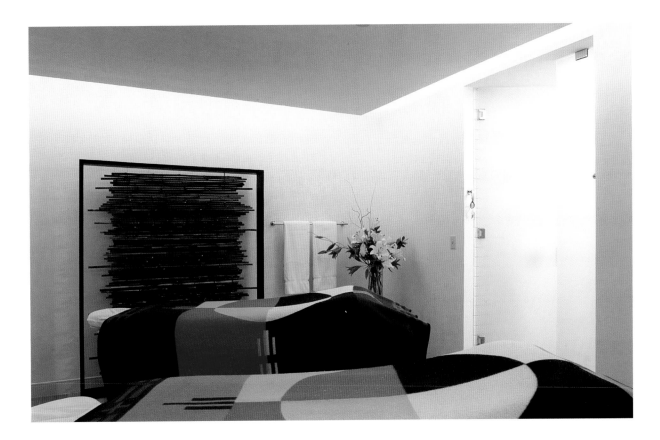

caveat emptor please, in acquiring suitable and relevant products only—and not the hype.

Nevertheless, be ever open to trying out new ingredients and new ways of looking at how your health is impacted by internal and external forces. And, be fearless in asking questions from different practitioners for a wider universe of responses to better understand new knowledge, as well as in getting satisfactory answers that make sense and are reasonable. And thanks to online search engines, accessing and reading up on information has never been easier.

Types of Spas

Many combinations, and different variations, of spa treatments spiced with Asian, Native American, and European flavors are constantly being developed, which makes it exciting for spa guests to return to sample them. There are, however, some operational differences.

Day spas do not offer overnight stays nor structured guest programs. They offer a variety of services such as manicures, pedicures, facials, massage and body work (dry and wet), and body

facing: This combination pool at Ojo Caliente revitalizes bathers with four natural springs bubbling into it.

The couple's treatment room at Nidah Spa, Eldorado Hotel, Santa Fe, New Mexico.

CHINESE CHI NEI TSANG

Never having had this treatment before, I was surprised when *Chi Nei Tsang* therapist Terri Picard at El Monte Sagrado Living Resort & Spa in Taos, began by explaining the Chinese concept of "beautifying the navel."

As I lay snug and draped on a portable treatment table in, appropriately, the China Suite, Picard identified the eight cardinal areas of *Chi Nei Tsang* (internal organ energy transformation). Radiating from the navel, they correspond to the body's major organs, such as north of the navel connecting the heart, and the left cardinal with the left kidney. Expertly massaging all eight cardinal areas to realign the navel's meridians for qi—the body's energy flow—to diffuse more efficiently, Picard added, "This also helps the body's lymphatic system eliminate toxins."

I was struck by the sublime, palpable feeling of being at total ease with the entire universe after being treated to *Chi Nei Tsang*. Was this a function of unclogging my meridians?

ANTI-AGING TIPS FOR LOOKING YOUNGER

Sergey Krupnov is a licensed aesthetician at The Spa at Mandarin Oriental Hotel, Washington D.C.

Krupnov's studies at St. Petersburg Medical University in Russia enabled him to develop an all-in-one facial-upper-body-back treatment that brings startling results. Beginning with upper body work followed by a facial, it unclogs energy meridians to facilitate body cells in metabolizing energy more efficiently—an altogether unique detoxification and relaxing treatment.

Here are some "Anti-Aging" tips from Krupnov to look and feel younger:

* Exercise daily if possible. Even a few minutes count in helping body cells metabolize oxygen intake more efficiently.
* Eat lots of fruits and vegetables. If possible, emphasize a plant-based diet with smaller portions of seafood or white meat. Periodically, abstain from eating meat for a week or two so your body can rest up from antibiotics and toxins in meat.
* Hydration is very important. Each person's requirement varies. Drink filtered or spring water as soon as you feel thirsty. Body cells plumped up with water will make skin look smoother, firmer, more luminous, and you therefore look younger.
* Have a facial at least once a month. Collagen and elastin, two proteins that contribute to skin elasticity, capture water more easily with facials stimulating blood circulation while detoxifying metabolic wastes from the cellular intake of oxygen.
* Be happy. Happiness is an important quality in looking younger. Positive energy impacts body cells by lessening stress—while worries, self-doubt, and suspicious energy makes a person look older.

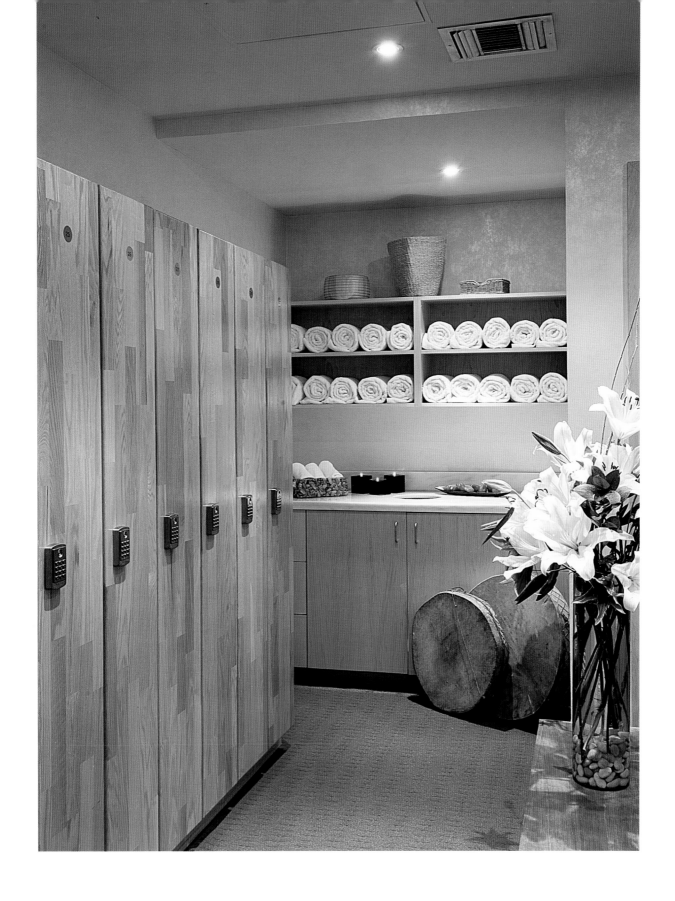

Natural accessories cast a soft glow in the
women's changing room at Nidah Spa,
Eldorado Hotel, Santa Fe, New Mexico.

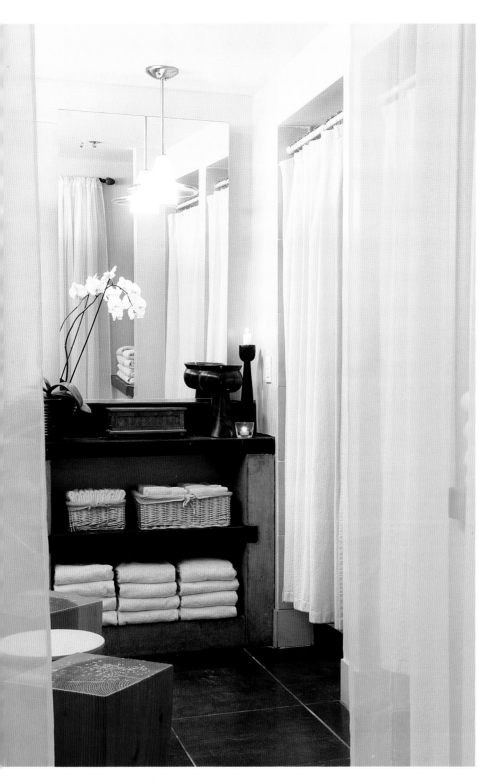

The women's changing room at ShaNah Spa at The Bishop's Lodge, Santa Fe, New Mexico.

wraps. Services typically are priced according to each session, ranging from twenty-five to fifty to eighty minutes, and many therapists are happy to accommodate special requests from guests.

Destination spas, however, require a stay of three to seven nights, in order for results to work out. (However temporary these results may be, they are nevertheless encouraging to discover, and continue to inspire newer aspirations of staying fit and beautiful, for good health's sake.)

The impact of destination spas, however, seems to last longer than the impact from day spas. The guest's extended immersion and unstinting attention from spa staff and the numerous activities they offer all work to focus and concentrate body, mind, and spirit in a total immersion of spa-related activities.

For instance, at Cal-a-Vie, guests check in with a counselor who quizzes them on their goals (such as weight gain or loss, muscle/joint flexibility and so on). Daily activities are then customized for each guest. The four core fitness components of this spa are cardiovascular (your aerobic capacity), strength training (for endurance), balance, and flexibility (in facilitating muscle and joint mobility). The same is true at other spas, as well.

Daily activities geared towards these fitness goals at Cal-a-Vie involve a hike over hill and vale every morning before breakfast, successively building in intensity and duration. After breakfast, other fun activities run the gamut of yoga to Pilates to salsa dancing. A mid-morning snack of

JAPANESE YASURAGI

Ten Thousand Waves Japanese Health Spa in Santa Fe is the only spa in the country offering nightingale facials. Duke Klauck, owner of The Waves, sources "the only nightingale poop facial cream factory left in Japan that pulverizes and purifies it for *geishas*, who have been using it to soften and whiten their faces," he says.

But I opted for a "non-poop" head and neck *yasuragi* massage that moisturizes and conditions the scalp with a warm concoction of camellia, rice bran, sesame, and jojoba oils. When twenty-five soothing minutes came and went, my scalp and body thirsted for more.

Luckily, this *sento*, or Japanese-style public bath, has a plethora of hot tubs—for men, women, communal, and private—where guests can extend their stay and continue soaking up and taking the waters (usually in the buff). Because water is the elixir of life that makes up two-thirds of the body, it just feels good to stay in any warm tub, any time.

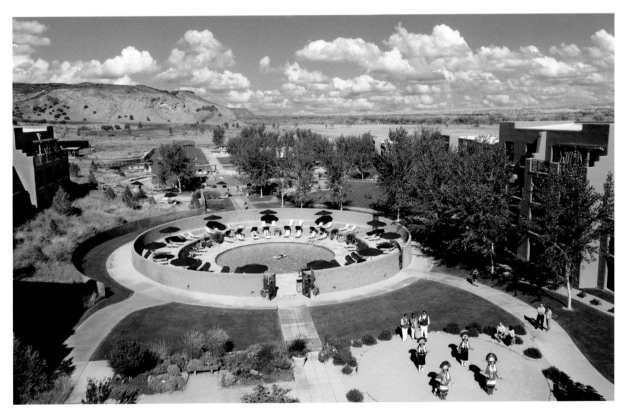

An aerial view of the gem-like setting of Tamaya Mist Spa & Salon on the grounds of the Hyatt Regency Tamaya Resort & Spa. (Photo courtesy Hyatt Regency)

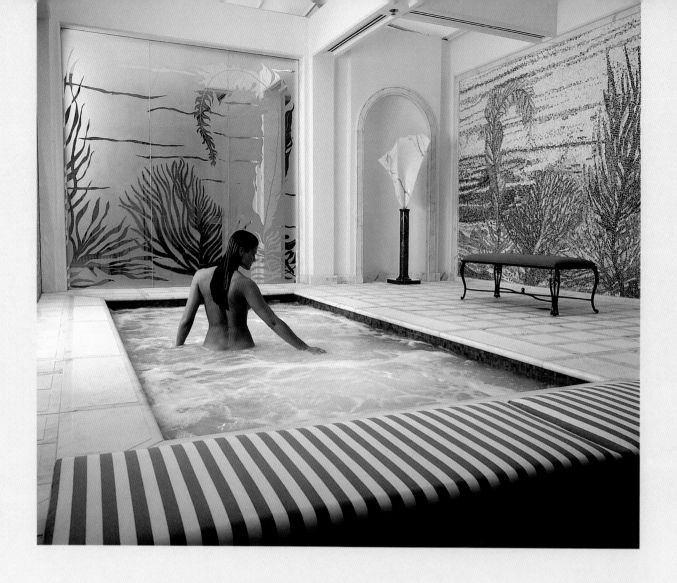

JAVANESE LULUR

The Javanese *lulur* oozes with an unparalleled treat for the body's senses. Since the seventeenth century, a Javanese bride-to-be is pampered forty days before her wedding with the *lulur*, a purifying ritual. Her body is anointed with the finest spices and yogurt, then tenderly massaged and bathed—resulting in exfoliated skin luxuriously soft to the touch.

The Inn at Loretto's SpaTerre in Santa Fe mixes warm yogurt with the traditional *lulur* paste of turmeric, ground rice, sandalwood, and jasmine. Gentle massage works in the paste together with warm honey. Afterwards, a steam shower stimulates yogurt cells to restore the skin's pH balance, while the honey nourishes and moisturizes the skin.

A well-trained masseuse leaves her imprint. In this case, Lynsey Rubin, of SpaTerre, identified six Javanese bodywork techniques she used. (1) With her knuckles, she deftly banished soreness from torso muscles and reenergized them. (2) While "wringing" the torso, she squeezed away stored-up stress. (3) My ribs delighted in rolling movements that peeled away exhaustion. (4) With both hands, Rubin "chopped away" tight tissue discomfort with karate-like, crisp chops. (5) The ankles got pulled down a few times and stre-e-e-tched for toes to touch the table. (6) Fingertips were "pulled off," by popping and loosening them. The entire *lulur* experience is an invigorating and fragrant one.

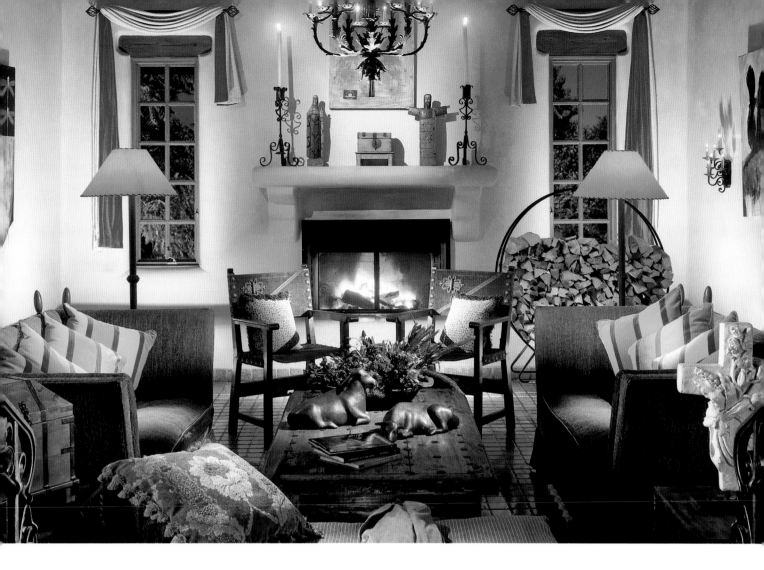

crudités and potassium broth[3] helps perk up energy levels before lunch on the patio.

The coup de grace of destination spas is their strategy of lavishing special treats with massages and facials to renew body and spirit in the afternoons. It's a strategy that works in rewarding efforts expended for the morning's rigorous and structured physical activities. It's also one that is easily adaptable at home— a workout first, followed by a luxuriously salubrious reward of your choice, on a regular basis.

Spa Services

The array of spa treatments that keep appearing with new dashes of local flavors can be mind-boggling and exciting to sample. Nidah Spa at Santa Fe's Eldorado Hotel works off a local gemstone by placing warm turquoise on the body's meridian points along the back as a signature touch to its Nidah Massage.[4] Across town at Avanyu Spa at La Posada de Santa Fe Resort, a delicious Chocolate Chipotle Wrap engulfs the senses and leaves guests salivating for more theobromic treats.

facing: Taking to the waters at Ihilani Resort and Spa on Oaʻhu Island in Hawaii. (Courtesy photo)

A warm welcome at the lobby of La Posada de Santa Fe Resort & Spa. (Courtesy photo)

[3] A similar Potassium Broth recipe from Golden Door spa is included in chapter 6, Enjoying Spa Cuisine.

[4] The spa's brochure says *Nidah* is a Native American word for "your life," but does not specify which Pueblo lingo it's from. There are nineteen independent Pueblos in New Mexico and other tribal nations such as the Navajo Nation.

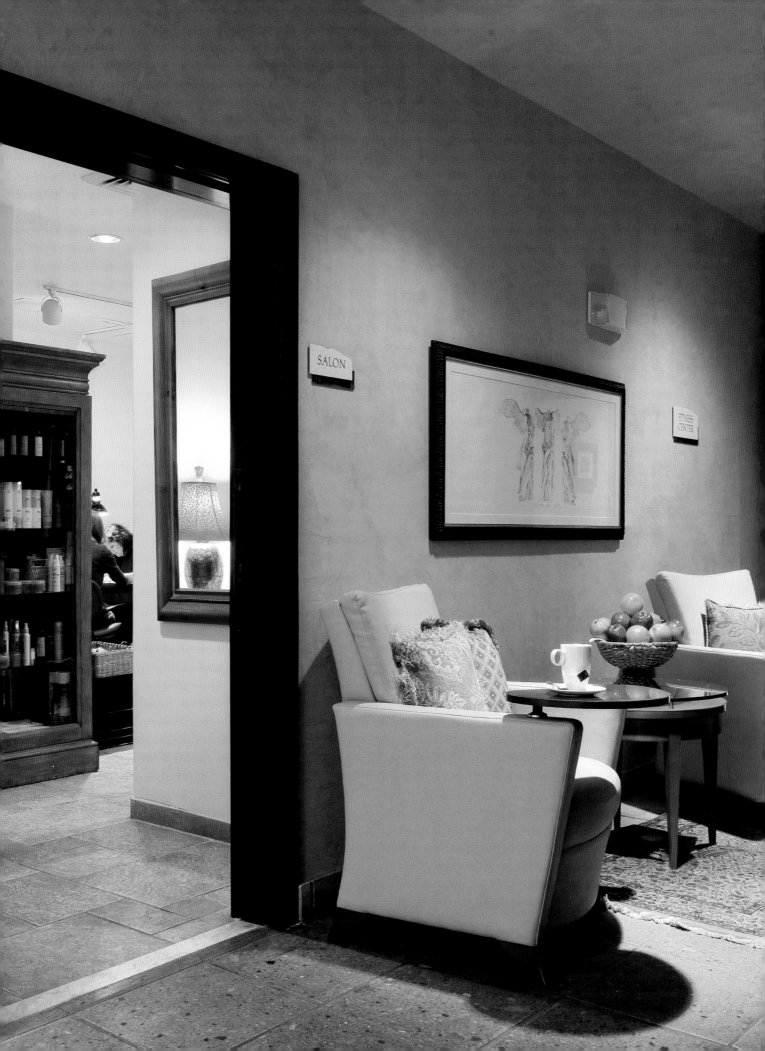

SALON

DESIGNING YOUR OWN SPA PROGRAM

It's easy to develop your own structured spa program at home. Although willpower and determination are more challenging for sticking with it, the rewards that come with a sense of well-being and an upbeat attitude are definitely worth the effort.

Below are four tips to getting started from Cal-a-Vie's checklist *How to Prepare for Your Cal-a-Vie Experience,* which primes guests to get more out of their stay.

1. *Start exercising.* Gradually get back into shape by walking, cycling, or swimming—not only for fitness sake, but for losing weight, as well. This happens because of the slow, steady burning of calories. Exercising at a medium intensity for a minimum of twenty minutes, and three times a week, will show results.

2. *Modify your diet.* Cal-a-Vie cuisine is low-fat and low-sodium, while high in complex carbohydrates such as whole grains, legumes, fresh vegetables, and fruits. For protein, fresh fish, turkey, free-range chicken, and tofu are served. Start introducing your palate to these foods while gradually cutting back the amount of fat, salt, and highly processed foods such as white sugar and white flour from your diet. Do this at least three weeks prior to your arrival. If you drink alcohol or smoke, try to cut down gradually (and go out for that walk instead).

3. *Drink ample water.* We encourage guests to drink eight to twelve, eight-ounce glasses of water a day to hydrate the body after exercise and to flush out waste products. Guests who are not used to this feel they have to answer the call of nature too frequently. It takes about a week for the bladder to adapt to fluid increases.

4. *See your doctor.* Please see your physician for a checkup before your arrival if you are over fifty, smoke, have not been exercising regularly, or have medical concerns.

facing: A calming cup of herbal tea revives the spirit in the cozy foyer of Avanyu (which means water serpent) Spa at La Posada de Santa Fe.

Native American accessories set the mood for a warm introduction to indigenous healing touches at ShaNah Spa, Santa Fe.

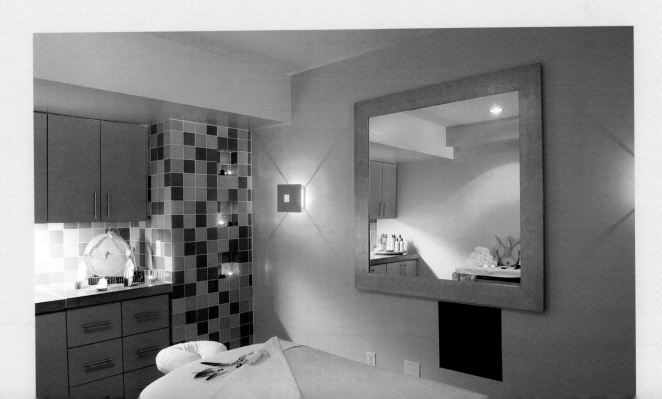

KOREAN-STYLE SPA AND BATHHOUSE

A Korean-style bathhouse and spa for women only at two locations north and south of Seattle "combines the traditional bath culture of Korea with the relaxation spa of today," says Sun Lee, general manager of Olympus Spa, which is owned by his parents, Mr. and Mrs. Myong Woon Lee.

Lee credits the Korean heating concept of *ohn-dol-bang* for six relaxation rooms that conduct warm energy more efficiently to maximize the body's metabolism. In fact, it was his father's gift to his mother who suffered from fevers and chills after the family emigrated to the wet, gray climate of Tacoma, Washington, in the 1990s. The first Olympus Spa opened there in June 1997. It was a source of consternation then, as neighbors were not used to hearing about nude women walking around inside the private spa area. But its healthy popularity as a healing sanctuary for women prompted the Lees to open another spa in 2005 north of Seattle, in Lynnwood, beside the convention center.

Olympus guests relax in six FIR (far infrared rays)[5] rooms—jade, mud with mugwort, oak charcoal, sand, elvan stone, and sea salt. Unlike direct solar energy, which burns the skin easily, FIR transmits energy by penetrating the skin on deeper levels, Lee says. When this happens, fat cells break down, body functions stabilize, blood pressure normalizes, and collagen production is activated; these are among some of the myriad health benefits Lee recounts in his information materials.

The aesthetic art of scrubbing the female anatomy and moisturizing services requires certification in Korea. Mrs. Lee is a certified instructor and trains all their therapists herself. Other regular spa beauty services such as facials are also offered. The Korean tea ceremony is a unique meditation arts practice. A separate Korean café adjoins it for an engaging all-day stay—resulting in a uniquely healing and aesthetic experience that encourages return visits.

But regardless of their delectably creative twists, from coast to coast, American spa services are generally divided into:

Massages

Most massages are a medley of the therapist's skills, ranging from deep-tissue Swedish-style[6] bodywork sans clothing, to Thai massage with guests fully clothed while being worked on.

Wraps

Skin is gently exfoliated before the body and head are covered cocoon-like in therapeutic mud wraps or thermal wraps that have been steeped in herbs, seaweed, or floral extracts. The herbs and mud are supposed to extract toxins from the body, as you lie blissfully prone for thirty to sixty minutes. Depending on the course of treatment, moisturizers are next applied on the skin to rejuvenate it.

An invitation to sunbathe at Tamaya Mist Spa & Salon. (Courtesy photo)

---

[5] FIR (far infrared rays) heating was discovered by German scientist Friedrich Wilhelm Herschel in spring 1800.

[6] A good online resource briefly describing Swedish massage and other areas of bodywork is at http://www.mamashealth.com/massage/sweed.asp.

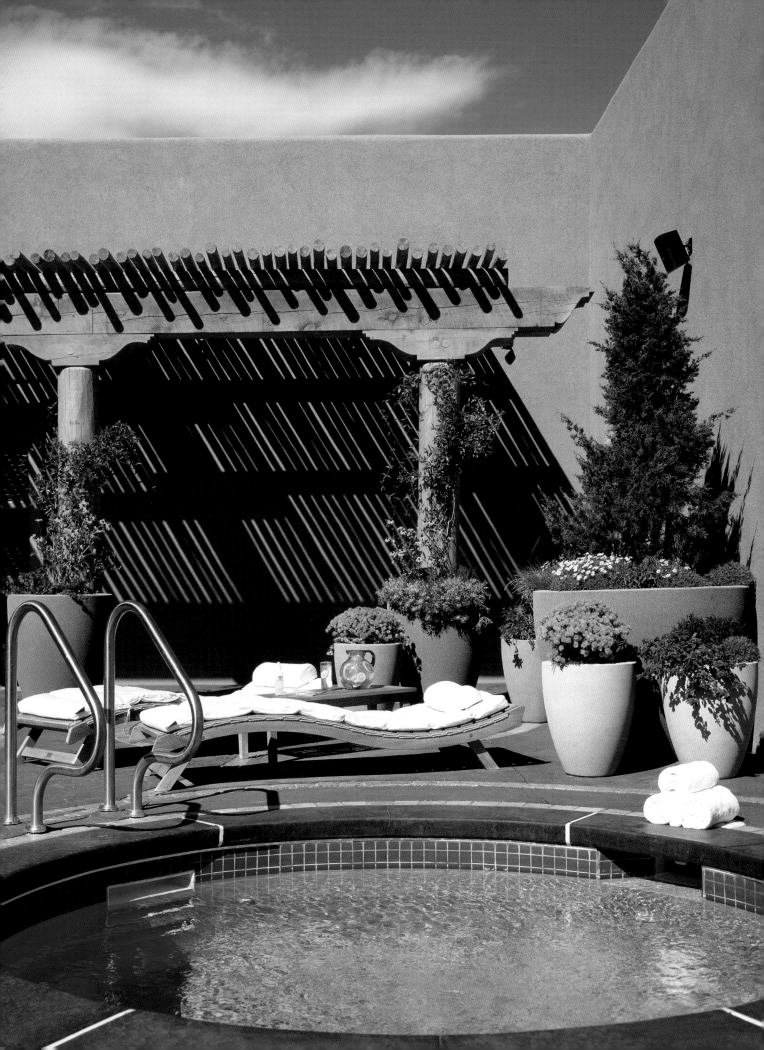

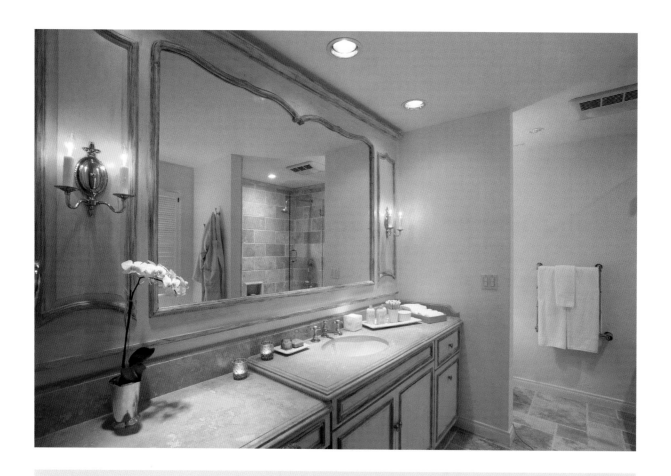

THE FINNISH SAUNA

No spa book is complete without mentioning the Finnish sauna as part of today's spa culture.[7] Christof Teuscher, a renowned scientist and author of books on Alan Turing (the father of modern computer science), grew up in Switzerland. His parents enticed him, his sister, and brother into the hot heat of a sauna (his dad liked to turn it up to 230 degrees Fahrenheit), with treats after each round of sauna "innings." It was a regular Saturday night feature for the family, culminating in the delicious fondue dinners the Swiss are known for, as everyone would be ravenous after the sauna sessions.

"We were always nude in the sauna. It was as natural as riding in a car for us kids," Christof

Teuscher recalls. Were his parents nudists or naturists? "Nope, we just had a very natural and healthy relationship with being nude," he says.

And that's something he and his wife, Ursina, share now too—even in the cold of winter. "One of my favorite moments of the hot sauna–cold plunge cycle is coming out of the plunge and lying down in the fresh, winter air," Ursina says, "and rolling around naked in the snow."

The Teuschers like to relax for about thirty minutes between each "inning," or round of sauna and cold plunges, and to drink lots of water. "It is not recommended that you go back into the sauna if you still feel hot," Christof cautions.

[7] Here is a fun introduction to taking the Finnish sauna: http://cankar.org/sauna/howto.html/

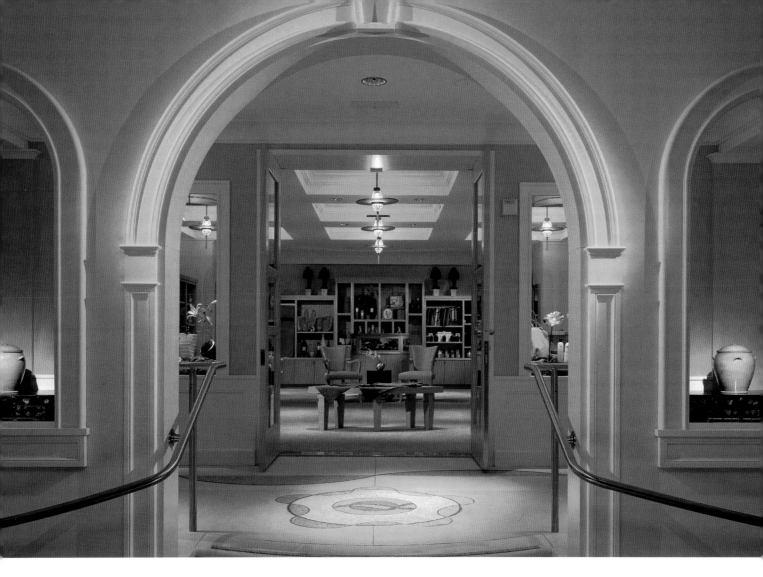

Scrubs

The body is first gently exfoliated of dead skin with a soft brush. Then an exfoliating paste (ranging from yogurt mixed with tropical spices, as in the Javanese *lulur*, to Dead Sea salts) is smeared over the body part that the therapist is simultaneously working on with techniques such as stretching the muscles and kneading muscle tissue with acupressure.

Facials

The aesthetician does a preliminary skin analysis first, and then uses the appropriate skin-care products to cleanse facial skin and exfoliate it of dermal debris. A masque is then applied to draw out toxins from the facial skin, and sometimes the aesthetician exits the room for the guest to lie in repose as the masque works its magic. The aesthetician then returns to peel away the masque, extract black heads, if needed, and finishes off by moisturizing the face and neck. Some aestheticians offer neck and shoulder massages—an altogether divinely luxurious treat!

facing: Cal-a-Vie's French-style stylish boudoir with mirrors bordered by carved silver-leafed frames encourages bathers to linger. (Courtesy photo)

The grand portal to Nob Hill Spa at The Huntington Hotel in San Francisco. (Courtesy photo)

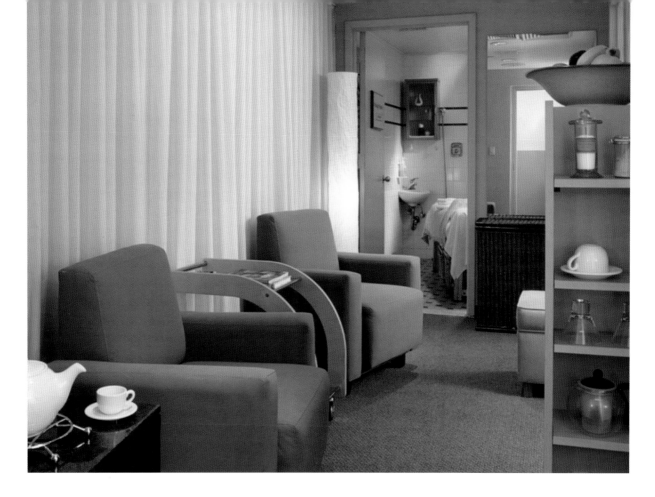

Other Beauty Services

These include foot reflexology, manicure, pedicure, waxing, and makeup and hair styling.

Lifestyle Services

Lifestyle coaching to expand the universe of healthy living options is commonly offered by destination spas, although a day spa like BODY of Santa Fe also offers them. These include nutrition counseling and even tarot-reading.

The onslaught of today's lifestyles can be so intense that we tend to get caught up in daily activities without realizing the need to renew with positive energy, and on a deeper level, to heal and recuperate. Spa services are designed to de-stress and revive—physically, emotionally, mentally, and spiritually.

This healing and rejuvenation is an excellent reason to incorporate spa visits, whether day or destination, into health-care routines—notwithstanding the fun and camaraderie shared with new acquaintances who invariably are easy to get to know because of similar aspirations for quality of life and living well.

Incidentally, some guests I've met at spas have shared their personal insights on these pages, to whom go heartfelt gratitude for their largesse, so others may be inspired by their experiences.

The waiting room at New York City's Parker Meridien Spa. (Courtesy photo)

facing: Arresting architecture at Cornelia Day Resort & Spa. (Courtesy photo)

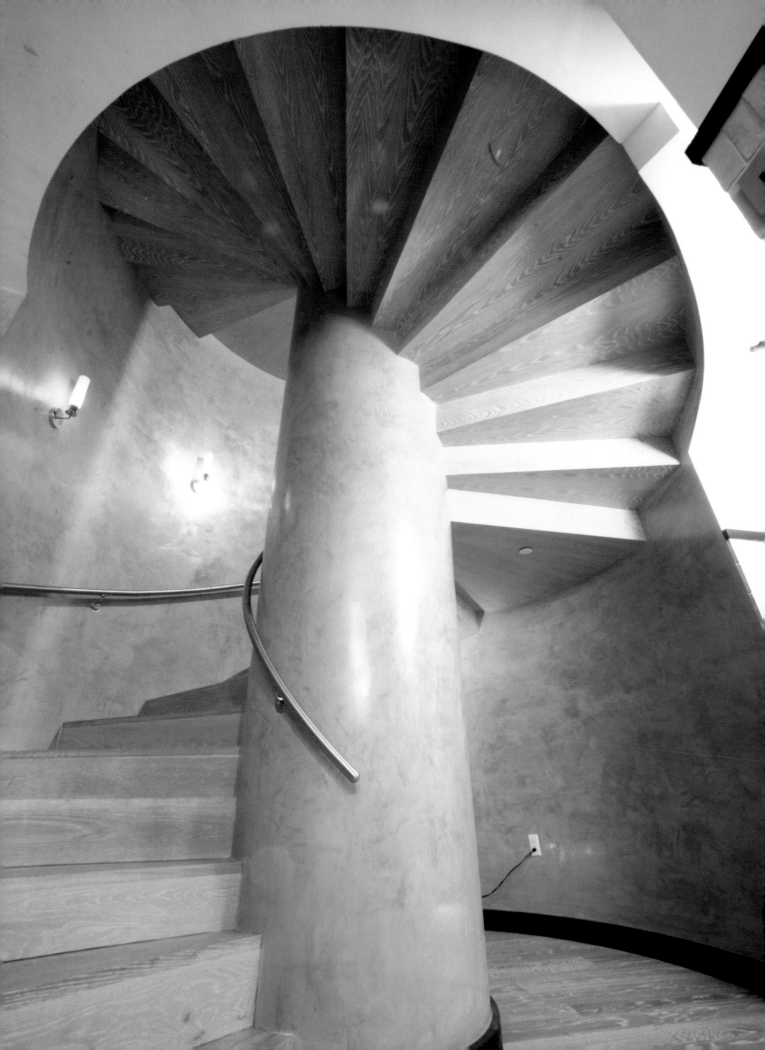

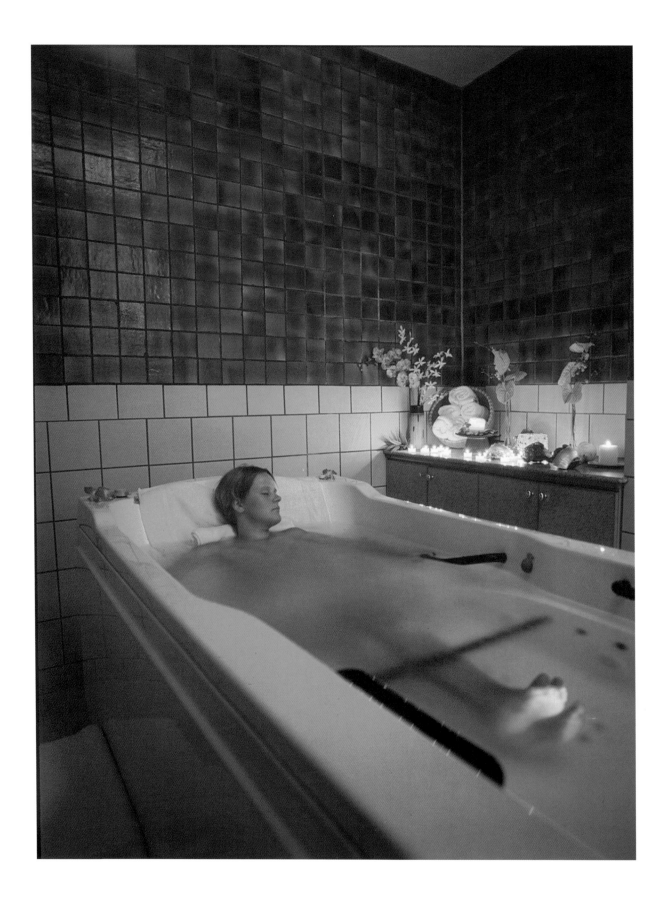

HOW I MELTED OFF FOUR AND A HALF INCHES THROUGH MY SEVEN-DAY STAY AT CAL-A-VIE

By Joan Messenger

I am still talking about my incredible lifestyle changes and experiences at Cal-a-Vie!

Getting up at 5:45 a.m. to go on a three- to five-mile hike every morning isn't anything I normally do. I found I enjoyed it though, and looked forward to it. Ever since, I have been going on a hike once a week. Our main home is in the Pacific Northwest, so we spent the summer hiking in the Cascades and Olympic mountains. My husband and adult children and their dogs go with me when it fits their schedule. I have continued my good exercise habits and have kept off the four and a half inches I lost while at Cal-a-Vie.

I arrived on a Saturday. When I checked in on Monday morning at the spa's fitness center, I was

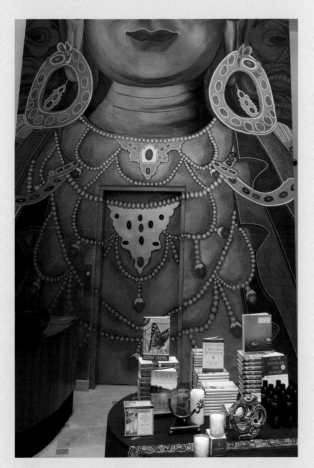

measured. I next met with the activities planner, who asked me how many calories I wanted to consume; together, we planned my daily activities for the week.

On the following Saturday, departure day, I was measured again and found I had lost four and a half inches! I lost one and a half inches off my waist, one inch off my hips, a half-inch off each thigh, and one inch off my chest, which was back fat.

I am now down a full size and my jeans are two sizes smaller (although not totally due to Cal-a-Vie, as I've kept up with my lifestyle changes). *I was not obese, so melting away four and a half inches in seven days is awesome!*

I do not keep up the 1,200-calorie spa diet, but I do watch what I am eating, and stick with a plan that works for me. I also work with personal trainers, do Pilates, plus hike for fun and exercise, ski, and golf every other day.

I found myself wondering how the great food served at Cal-a-Vie stayed within the 1,200-calorie diet I chose.[8] Chef (Steve Pernetti) was very helpful and gave me recipes that were not in Cal-a-Vie's first cookbook. I enjoyed the cooking demonstrations and have implemented some of his recipes into my own cooking.

I have signed up to go again next year and invited some friends to go with me. I am making Cal-a-Vie an annual event.

facing: **Taking to the waters with color thalasso therapy at Ihilani Resort and Spa. (Courtesy photo)**

The colorful frescoed foyer to the Chopra Center & Spa at Dream, New York City. (Courtesy photo)

[8] As an example of how spas customize guest needs, this book's author was put on an 1,800-calorie diet, which she reduced to 1,200 calories subsequently. See the bibliography for a selected list of spa cookbooks.

MELTING THE ICE, SPA STYLE

By Joan Messenger

(Note: There is something quite inexplicable about dropping our defenses while working on self-improvement along with others who are also trying hard, each in our own way. A serene spa ambiance is a soothing counterpoint to guests animatedly swapping ideas and stories.)

There was a gal from New York who said she was an interior designer and had been to every spa in the U.S. and some in Europe. She was as tight as a tick when she came in. I mentioned that I had read Cal-a-Vie was the best spa as it is small, with a high ratio of staff to clients. Also, I had had a chance to talk to the previous week's guests as they were leaving while I was checking in. They were all thrilled with their experiences.

This designer responded in very chilly tones, "I'll let you know at the end of the week." So I decided I did not want to sit with her again after that first Sunday's dinner.

But by the end of the week, she was a different person. We sat with each other at meals, chatting like old friends! She said she had saved the best for last, and would be back in two months.

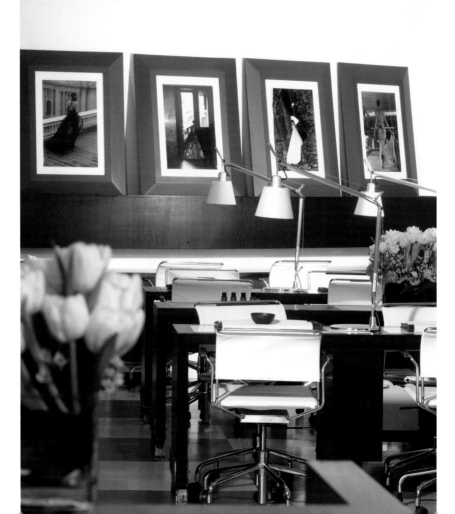

A touch of haute at the manicure room at Cornelia Day Resort & Spa. (Courtesy photo)

facing: A full body massage after a gym workout at The Westin at Times Square. (Courtesy photo)

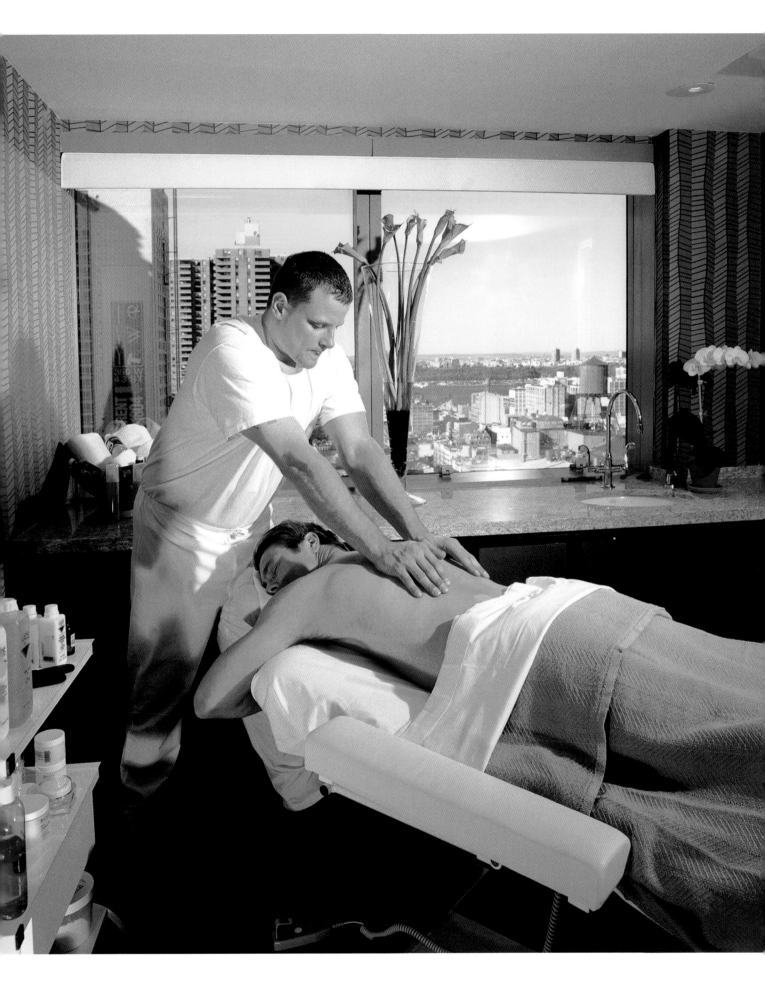

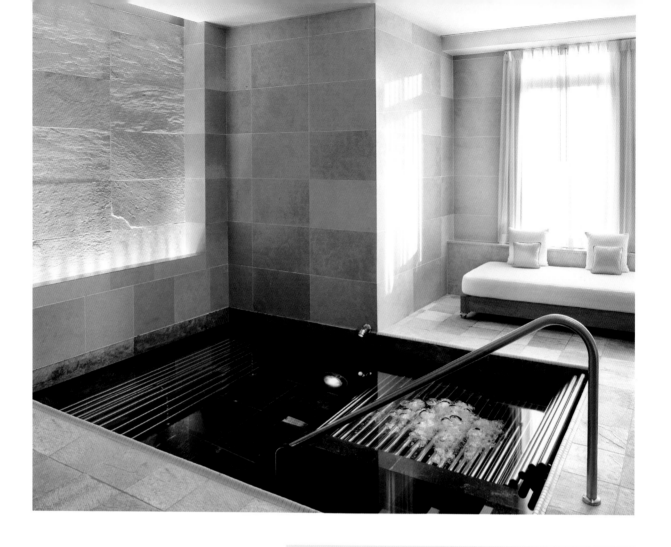

The vitality pool gently restores energy at New York's Mandarin Oriental Spa. (Courtesy photo)

facing: Blissing out at the Palm Springs Parker Meridien Spa in California. (Courtesy photo)

THE WORLD OF WATER HEALTH

While Americans enjoy the luxury of bathing in their own bathrooms, many cultures around the world take to public baths. Either because of the lack of a bathroom at home (still the case in many less developed countries and even in some cramped living spaces in Japan's urban cities where space is at a premium and the tradition of taking baths at the *sento* continues) or historical habits and the preference for communal bathing, the culture of the bath is still very much alive today.

Jane Brenton's masterful translation of *The Book of the Bath* (Rizzoli, 1998) by Francoise de Bonneville is a wondrous rendition of bath cultures around the world, from the Turkish *hammam* to the Russian *banya*, among others. With water as a symbol of purification and the source of health and regeneration coursing through this book, aqueous histories and cultures appeal with an innate intimacy.

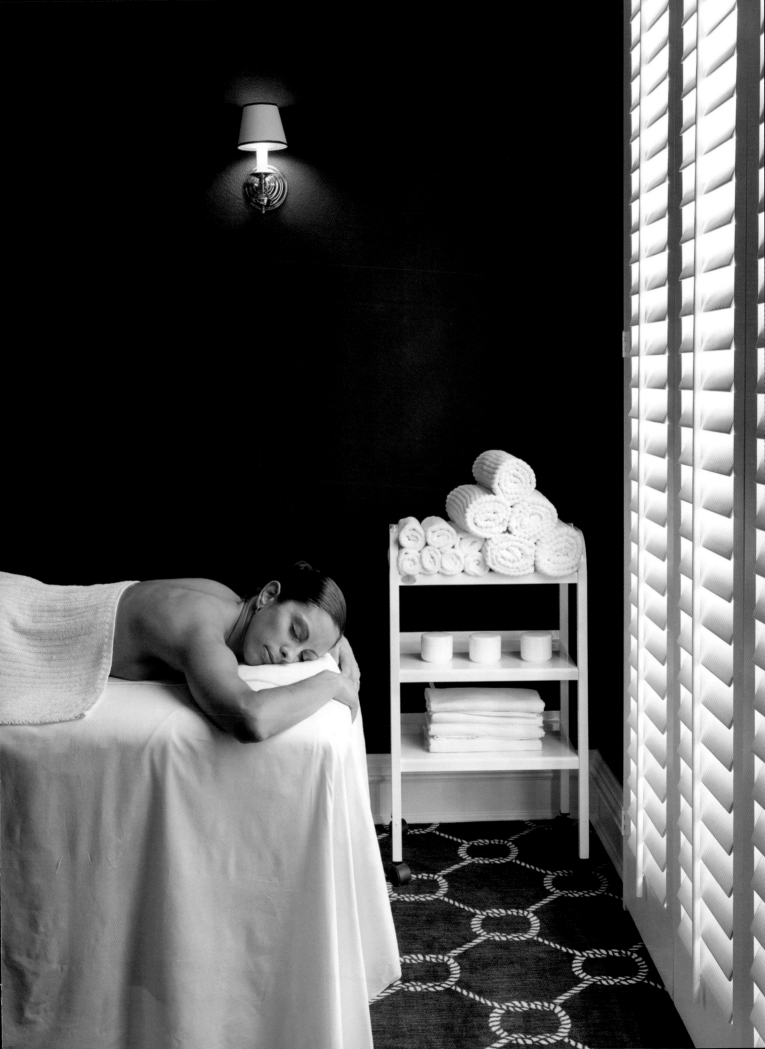

CHAPTER THREE

INCORPORATING PROPER SKIN CARE

It's quite amazing! When a person is of sound mind, body, and spirit, they have a very distinct glow. It is extremely important to take time to pamper yourself. It is no longer a luxury, but rather, a healthy necessity.

—Hippo Lipkin, Spa Director, Mandara Spa Hawaii, LLC, Hilton Hawaiian Village, Honolulu, Hawaii

With her cutting-edge book, *Absolute Beauty: Radiant Skin and Inner Harmony through the Ancient Secrets of Ayurveda* (Harper Perennial, 1997), New York City aesthetician Pratima Raichur opened new doors to both looking at, and achieving, beauty. Raichur describes beauty as "the pure energy of consciousness . . . a profound experience of wholeness . . . an effortless poise, grace, and vibrance: the individual totally at ease from *deep within the skin* and radiant from without."[1]

More importantly, Raichur drives home the point that without happiness, lasting beauty is an unattainable goal. It is only when harmony of body, mind, and spirit is present that natural beauty presents the gift of good health to a person, in tangible and holistic ways.

It's a healthy echo in the Southwest too. Kim Telles, manager of Tamaya Mist Spa and Salon at the Hyatt Regency Tamaya Resort and Spa in Santa Ana Pueblo, New Mexico, notes, "Spa trends are moving more toward wholeness—meaning, spas are taking the person as a whole and creating treatments and packages according to their lifestyles."

For, as an innovative heart physician has shown in his book, *Dr. Dean Ornish's Program for Reversing Heart Disease* (Ballantine, 1996), it is possible to regain good health by modifying a person's diet, as well as adopting positive lifestyle changes such as exercise and meditation to promote healing. Additionally, the divine element of love—including unconditionally forgiving self and others—is "real medicine" that heals too, Ornish wrote in his later book, *Love and Survival* (HarperCollins, 1998).

Natural clay facials exfoliate and cleanse, for skin to feel soft again at SpaOlakino, Honolulu. (Courtesy photo)

---

[1] Page 8. Raichur's first chapter, "What Is Beauty?" is a wealth of intriguing information.

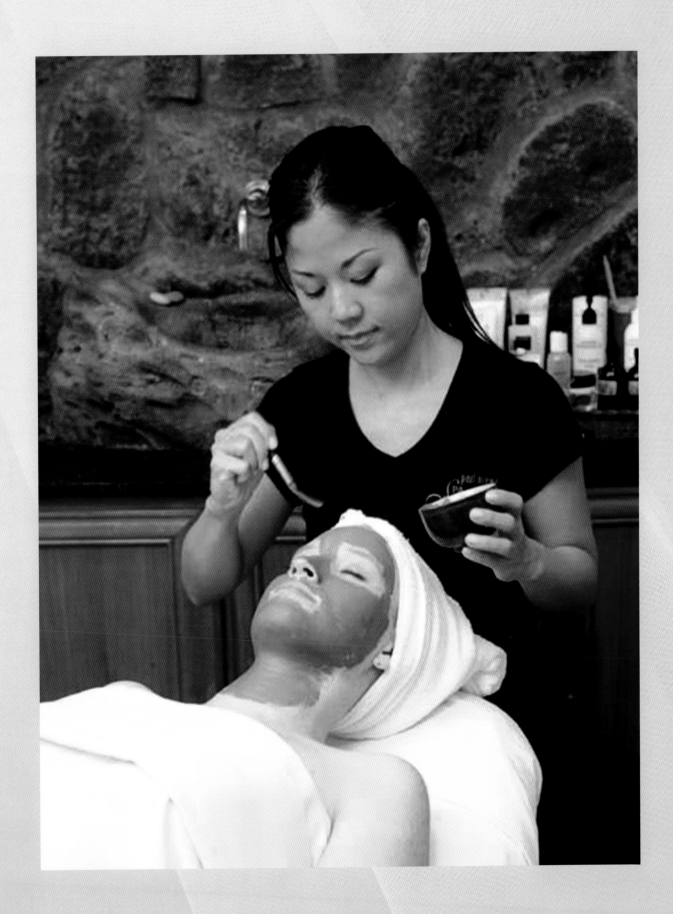

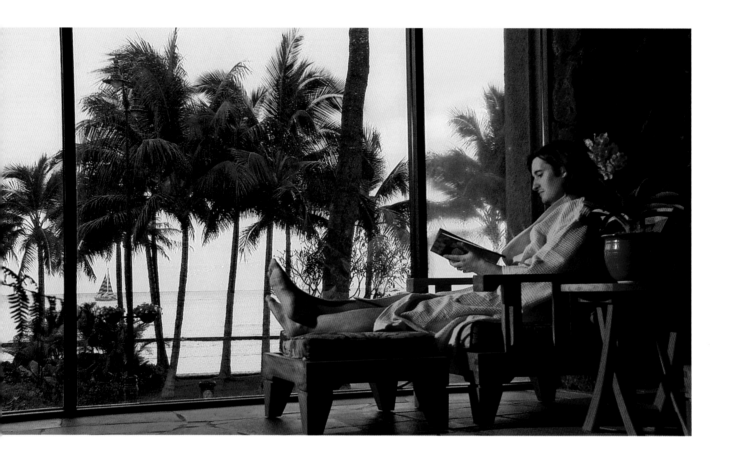

Relaxing with views of Waikiki Beach after a spa treatment at SpaOlakino in Honolulu. (Courtesy photo)

facing: Spices are integral to Indonesian-style spa treats, as dished up at Absolute Nirvana Spa in Santa Fe, New Mexico.

Facial Skin Care for Health and Beauty

Gabrielle Wagner, a Santa Fe, New Mexico, aesthetician with over half a century's distillation of skin-care education and experience, tells of a successful business owner who wanted to present "a new face" at her board meeting. After Wagner finished this person's facial, she immediately noticed how at ease this woman was—to the point where her deep wrinkles had eased out smoothly, and that she actually looked less wrinkled—thus illustrating vividly the mind-body connection affecting a person's makeup.

Wagner offers priceless nuggets of beauty secrets and advice that make women beautiful from having worked on three continents: first in her native Germany, later in Australia, and in the United States since 1999.

She helps women discover that true beauty is, ultimately, radiance from within, defined by a flash of inner knowing that radiates from the person's core of self-confidence—a confidence born of cherishing their own uniqueness.

FACIAL SKIN *IS* AN AGENT OF ELIMINATION

By Gabrielle Wagner, Aesthetician and Owner, JURLIQUE of Santa Fe, New Mexico

The healthy body functions well while assimilating good food with regular elimination. Similarly, the facial skin is nourished by nutrients transported to it via the lymphatic system, and the need to eliminate dead cells from it.

1. It is not helpful to rub and scrub the facial skin to rid it of impurities (as this presses them deeper inside)—which only results in clogging the pores and stretching the delicate skin surface to create even more wrinkles.

2. Instead, bathe and soak your face in warm water using a washcloth to prepare the skin for proper cleansing.

3. Next, wash your face by spreading the cleanser over your wet hands and applying it with a press-and-release motion, to impact the skin on a deeper level, which not only removes the surface dead skin cells, but also activates the lymph function of releasing toxins from within. Use lots of water during this process.

4. Finish by compressing your skin with a washcloth soaked in cold water, to tone and tighten your skin.

5. For the day, moisturize your clean skin liberally with an organic rosewater or herbal toner, followed by a cream, lotion, or oil for protection. Do this before applying makeup, and sunscreen with UVA/UVB protection if you will be out and about.

6. After thorough cleansing, rest your skin at night with a nourishing liquid or gel, instead of creams, to aid the skin's self-repair while sleeping.

7. Always be gentle with your facial skin and it will glow at any age!

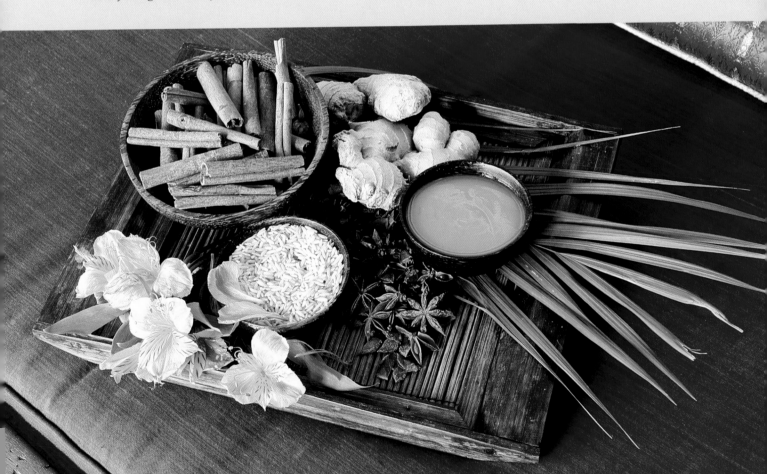

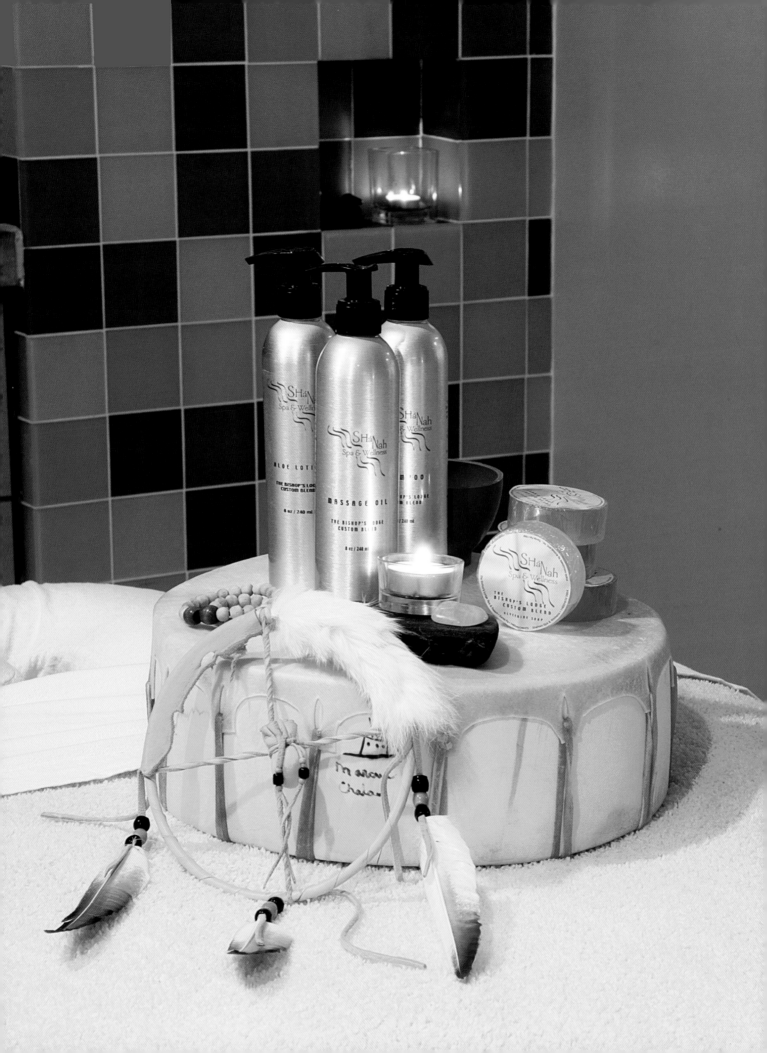

"This inner confidence takes time to cultivate—as do the botanical products I use, which are harvested according to nature's own rhythms, and then processed for many months. The prolonged process first releases their true essences while preserving the plants' life force, before [they are] formulated as skin-care products," Wagner explains.

"And, the final product is much more potent than individual plant parts," Wagner claims, "in revitalizing, nourishing, and protecting your skin without the use of petrochemicals." She believes the important point to be wary about is how some large cosmetic corporations extract certain plant parts without using the whole plant to achieve an overall synergy invaluable to human application.

Early on, Wagner had been training aestheticians for the organic line of German cosmetics called Dr. Hauschka. In 1985, Dr. Jurgen Klein, an alchemist and naturopath, and his wife, Ulrike, a botanist and horticulturalist, hired Wagner to train aestheticians in the San Francisco Bay Area to use their new natural skin-care products, JURLIQUE.

Ever since, Wagner has been trying to instill in women the fact that true beauty transcends age, culture, and social expectations. Whenever a client is doubtful about her appearance, Wagner suggests she asks herself three questions:

- Why am I doing this to myself?
- Why am I trying to change myself to suit other people's expectations and preferences (especially when dating)?
- What could happen if I take the time, and care for my skin, just for myself?

Having practiced on three continents, Wagner is struck by disparities in cultural perceptions. In Europe, women use makeup in a more discreet way. In fact, she laughingly adds, call girls use heavier makeup as their calling card.

In the United States, she sees women generally using lots more makeup, probably in response to media hype, peer pressure, and/or spousal influences in admiring women on television and in the movies as their beauty ideal.

Wagner finds too, that European women perceive the role of aesthetics differently—in regarding skin care as a preventive daily ritual vital to restoring and maintaining the skin's naturally healthy state. Whereas, in the United States, women are only just now beginning to understand the value of using natural cosmetics and seeing the benefits of professional facials on a regular basis.

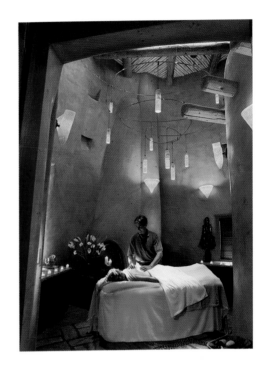

facing: Spa products specially formulated for ShaNah Spa at The Bishop's Lodge, Santa Fe, New Mexico.

It's easy to drift away in an adobe treatment room at El Monte Sagrado Living Resort & Spa. (Courtesy photo)

THREE AYURVEDIC BEAUTY RECIPES

by Sonia Elisa Masocco
Instructor, The Ayurvedic Institute,
Albuquerque, New Mexico

Most of the ingredients in these
recipes are available at health food
stores or from:
www.fromnaturewithlove.com.

Fragrant Facial Nutritive Mask
(*tridoshic*)

2 tablespoons colloidal oatmeal
(superfine regular oatmeal ground in
blender)
2 teaspoons goat milk powder
1/2 teaspoon multani mitti clay (yellow
clay from India, which can be substituted with plain white kaolin clay)
1 teaspoon rose petal powder
1 teaspoon sandalwood powder
2 drops rose attar (essential rose oil from
India infused in a sandalwood base)

Mix all dry ingredients in a small jar
with a tight-fitting lid. Take half of the
dry powder and mix in one ounce of
warm water; to this, add one drop of
rose attar. (The amount of water may
vary depending on humidity levels of
the region—just be sure you have a
consistency that spreads easily). It is
now ready to be applied either by
brush, or with the fingers. Allow the
application to remain on the skin for
fifteen to twenty minutes before rinsing
off with warm water.

continued

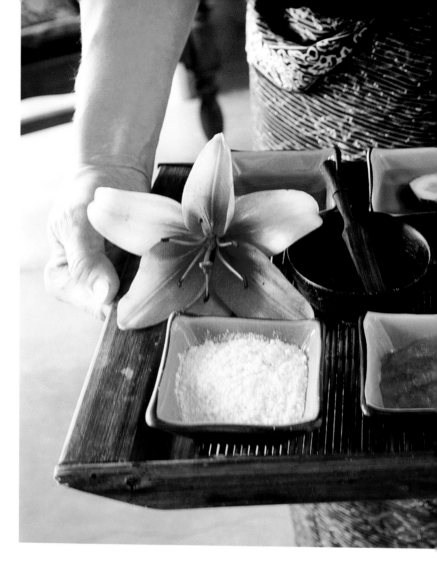

"In going beyond outer beauty, women have to learn that
they cannot indefinitely hide their skin and their persona behind
masks of makeup, but instead learn to appreciate, love, and celebrate their own unique features," Wagner advises.

Indeed, each individual is created as uniquely as each flower
and snowflake is. Many astute aestheticians use a combination of
organic beauty products from different product lines to achieve
radiant results for their clients. An even more customized
approach is adopted in Ayurveda beauty care, the herbal science
of skin care from India.

"Ayurveda is the doorway to deeper, inner beauty," enthuses
Sonia Elisa Masocco, who teaches Ayurvedic Beauty Concepts at
The Ayurvedic Institute[2] in Albuquerque, New Mexico. It is a
beauty that answers to no stereotypes. "True beauty is from
within—not cosmetically nor surgically applied from the outside,"
Masocco emphasizes. Instead, the body's largest organ, the skin,
plays a major role in revealing the person's internal state of health.

"It's like you're making your own movie and starring in it by
showcasing your unique beauty that's different from everyone

[2] The Ayurvedic Institute (www.ayurveda.com) was founded by Dr. Vasant Lad in 1984. It is recognized as one of the preeminent Ayurvedic schools and treatment facilities outside of India.

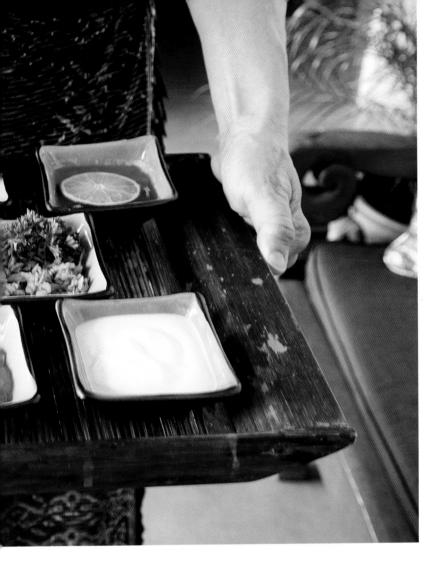

else's," Masocco says. "How so? By the person being empowered to address food and lifestyle changes to reduce physical stress afflicting their body and mind. They're free to be happy, and be completely at ease with who they truly are," she adds.

"The primary advantage of Ayurvedic beauty care is the ability to call your own shots—by assessing your skin's present condition, eating foods that balance your dosha, or constitutional type, making smart lifestyle adjustments, and customizing facial and beauty-care products for your own skin type to rebalance for natural healing, as well as bringing out your inner radiance," says Masocco.

There are three doshas: *vata* (the energy of movement), *pitta* (the energy of digestion and metabolism), and *kapha* (the energy of lubrication). Although a person's constitution is governed by one or two dominant dosha(s), the body needs all three types of energy to be balanced for optimum health.

"The principles of Ayurveda are really quite simple—where like increases like, and opposites balance out," Masocco advises. "So, for example, if you're a *pitta*, which governs the energy of

Almond Milk Cleanser (*tridoshic*)

20 whole almonds
1 cup water
2 ounces rose hydrosol or lavender hydrosol
4 drops geranium essential oil
1 ounce vegetable glycerine

Soak the almonds overnight and peel them. Blend in blender with the water and until liquefied; strain to remove residuals. Add the hydrosol to the almond milk, then the geranium essential oil, and then the vegetable glycerine. Shake vigorously before use. If kept refrigerated in an airtight container, this cleanser can last up to two weeks.

Ubtan (*tridoshic exfoliant/scrub*)

1 part rice bran powder
1 part chickpea powder
1/4 part hibiscus powder
1/4 part rose powder
1/4 part sandalwood powder
1/4 part coriander powder

Mix the ingredients together. When ready to use, take the amount needed and add a few drops of water to moisten before applying with circular movements to face and neck.

Note: *tridoshic* makes it applicable to all types of dosha.

Serving up a tropical-style facial treat at Absolute Nirvana Spa in Santa Fe, New Mexico.

79

digestion and metabolism, you're more prone to dynamic heat. You'd want to park your car in the shade, wear a hat, and drive about later in the evening or earlier in the morning to avoid the sun's more powerful rays in the middle of the day."

Daily habits either balance or imbalance the body, with continuous detrimental actions hurting the body (such as stress from meeting constant deadlines and pulling successive all-nighters) to result in six stages of imbalance that burden the body with less than perfect health.

Masocco says the first three stages are easier to arrest with modifications to diet and lifestyle—accumulation, provocation, and spreading the imbalance to vulnerable tissue areas (which have been prone to previous injury) that manifest in breakouts such as acne, rash, eczema or even dryness (as in dry joints and dry skin). Often, while the person may feel out of sorts and outer symptoms have not manifested, medical science may not have a diagnosis for it, yet.

According to Masocco, the fourth, fifth, and sixth stages are more complicated and require professional attention from a trained Ayurvedic practitioner to detoxify and purify the body. Once the body tissue has been invaded, the accumulated doshas, or energies, lodge in as unwelcome squatters, leading to the fifth stage of imbalance by multiplying aggressively. The sixth stage is secondary pathogenesis.

The Ayurvedic Institute's Panchakarma Program helps patients cleanse and heal with herbs during their three-, five-, or seven-day stays. *Pancha* means five, while *karma* means action. It is a detoxifying program that involves the five basic elements of nature: ether, air, fire, water, and earth.

Manicure and pedicure treatments amidst the fabled grandeur of a Mughal setting at the Chopra Center & Spa at Dream, New York City. (Courtesy photo)

HYDROSOLS

by Sonia Elisa Masocco

Hydrosols are by-products of the steam distillation of essential oils. They have almost a homeopathic dosage of the essential oil constituents, and cost less than essential oils. Similar to hydrosols are floral waters to which essential oil drops have been added to water. A typical floral water consists of eight drops of a high to medium note (such as lemon and lavender) or four drops of a medium to base note (such as rose, geranium, or sandalwood) added to four ounces of purified water.

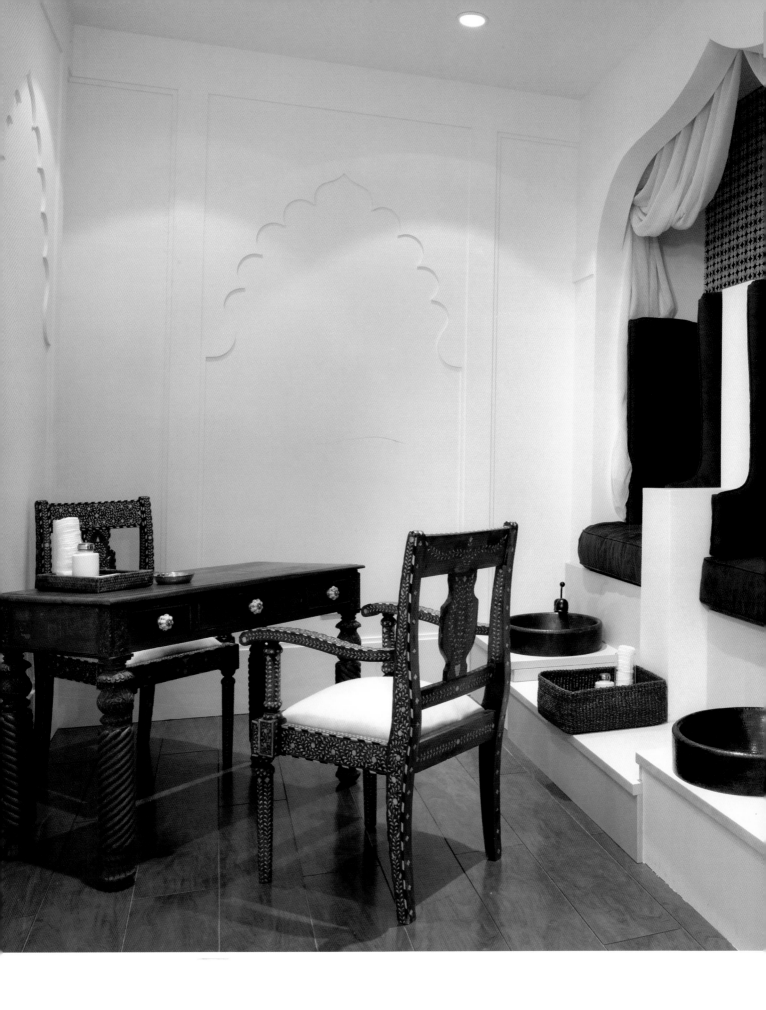

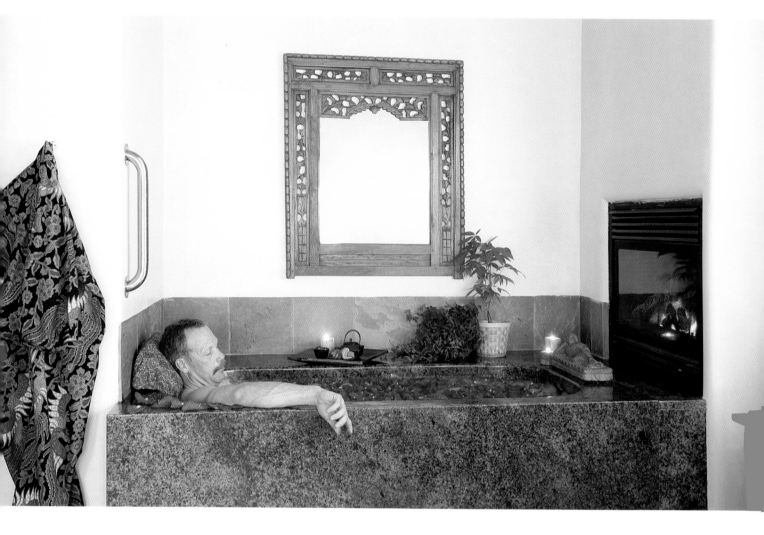

Many men are discovering and luxuriating in spa amenities such as this rose-petal soak at Absolute Nirvana Spa in Santa Fe, New Mexico.

"Best of all, Ayurveda is an empowering healing science and a conscious art of beautiful living where a person can have total control of their actions that affect their well-being, even as they are responsible for their own actions," Masocco offers.

Skin Care for Men

Increasingly, men are enjoying facials and honing up on good skin-care practices. "I'm glad to see more men coming to Miraval Spa," reports resident acupuncturist Donald Kimon Lightner. "Men have to learn to take care of themselves. Spa treatments are not just 'fluff and buff,' but can mitigate health concerns before they become too serious to handle. Spa treatments are not just 'girly' activities—but are fun, purifying, and health-oriented—guys need to rebalance their mind, body, and spirit, as well," urges Lightner.

THE NPD GROUP REPORTS MEN'S
PRESTIGE SKINCARE SALES CAN GROW TO $1 BILLION.[4]

"Men are starting to embrace the concept of taking care of their skin beyond washing it with bar soap," said Karen Grant, senior beauty analyst at The NPD Group, in her online press release. "The products that we see in the prestige market that are doing well are those that are simple and multipurpose, products that are part of a basic regimen, like cleansers, moisturizers, and shave treatment products."

Men's moisturizers and treatment shave represent 51 percent of the men's total prestige skin-care sales. These two sub-segments combined had a total of $16.3 million in sales for the first half of 2006. Facial exfoliators ranked third among men's sub-segments with $3.7 million in sales. Facial cleansers ranked fourth with double-digit growth of 14 percent in the first six months of this year versus last year and sales totaled $3.4 million.

"Sales of men's prestige skin-care products (sold in U.S. department stores) for the first half of 2006 reached $32 million, up 3 percent from the same time in 2005. It continues to grow at a time when women's prestige skin-care sales are flat for 2006," the release stated.

While hovering at $70 million for the year, Grant sees an opportunity for this new market segment for men's upscale skin-care sales to tip the $1 billion mark.

But interestingly, men pay 46 percent or $16 less on average for prestige skin-care products—$18.56 in the first half of 2006 (up 3 percent from last year), while the average price women spend on prestige skin care for the same period was $34.53.

(Note: An inverse correlation worth pondering, in comparing male-female earnings on the job, where women are generally paid about 25 percent less on average.)[5]

"Some of the deeper life issues [for both men and women] that emerge in guests who undergo acupuncture sessions with me are frustration at goals that were perhaps impeded, anger at not having demands met, and depression. These feelings manifest in the physical as lower and upper back pain, shoulder aches, headaches, insomnia, menstrual problems, and even infertility," Lightner adds.

Depending on the individual, Lightner administers a combination of acupuncture or acupressure with Chinese herbal remedies. Clients are encouraged to continue seeking similar services upon returning home. There is a wealth of spa healing practices that work their magic differently on individuals, men, or women.

Hippo Lipkin, Mandara Spa director in Honolulu, also urges men to consider skin care as an important grooming and health

[4] October 19, 2006, from an online press release at http://www.npd.com/press/releases/press_061019.html.

[5] "Gender Pay Gap, Once Narrowing, Is Stuck in Place," David Leonhardy, *New York Times*, December 24, 2006.

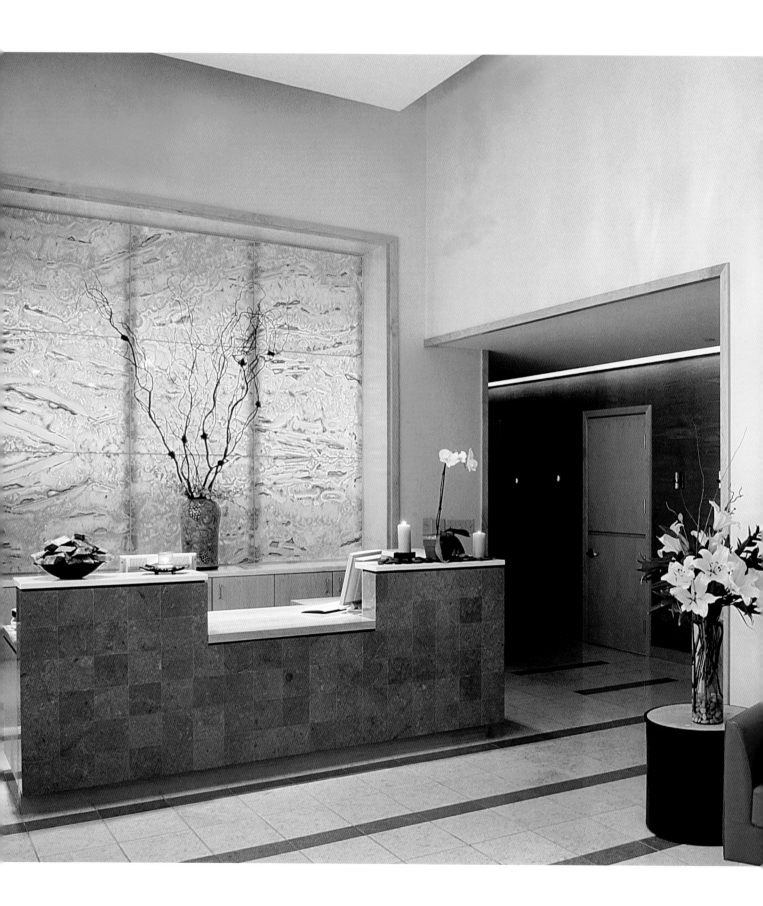

habit. "I think most men do not look after their skin, as we tend to think it's 'a lady's thing.' But in fact, we do have to take as much care for clear, healthy-looking skin that reflects our internal state of health," advises Lipkin. He has a facial once a week, using their in-house botanical-based Elemis face scrub. Daily use of Elemis shaving cream helps too, as he finds it gives him a better shave and makes his skin feel, and look, better.

Gary Rohana, spa director at Honolulu's SpaOlakino, suggests, "Guys should take the time to learn about their skin type and what daily routines and products work best for them. Their aesthetician or dermatologist is a good source for advice. Many guys make the mistake of using products suggested by their girlfriend, wife, or mom. Why? Because there is no one item that works for everyone. And, avoid overexposure to the sun even though you may have slathered on sunscreen that has UVA and UVB protection."

He points out that ingrown facial hair follicles can sometimes be very irritating for guys. "There are products and medications that can address serious ingrown hair issues, but for minor cases, regular light-moderate exfoliation will help the hair find the skin's surface—another good reason to cleanse, exfoliate, and moisturize your skin daily," Rohana likes to remind his clients.

"I struggled with ingrown hair for years, and thought it was normal, and nothing could be done. Boy, was I wrong!" says Dan Mohr, spa director of Avanyu Spa at La Posada de Santa Fe. "There are two important aspects to controlling ingrown hairs— proper shaving techniques and keeping the skin well hydrated. My shaving routine starts with applying a pre-shave oil to the freshly cleansed face to soften the beard (a pre-shave oil with an essential oil such as lemon or other citrus is a nice 'waker-upper').

"Next, a shaving cream without alcohol is important to avoid drying out the skin. (I personally like products from The Art of Shaving). Using a razor with fresh, sharp blades, always shave with the direction the beard grows—most important. After a cool rinse, use a high-quality moisturizer, such as Phytomer's 'Homme' line. I haven't had any ingrown hair since starting this routine," notes Mohr.

At the Golden Door spa in Escondido, California, Andrea Miller, who develops and manages the spa's specialty skin-care product line, explains that ingrown hairs occur when new hair growth cannot break through the skin and therefore starts

ENHANCING YOUR IMMUNE SYSTEM FOR HEALTHY SUN CONSCIOUSNESS

By Gabrielle Wagner,
Aesthetician and Owner,
JURLIQUE of Santa Fe,
New Mexico

With the ozone layer thinning, we are even more challenged by the sun. But, instead of living in ignorance or trying to outsmart nature with chemical applications, wouldn't it be more beneficial for us to develop a respectful relationship with the sun, and to use our intelligence to befriend this wondrous source of life-giving energy?

Shouldn't we instead build up our faces and bodies with good nutrition to enhance our immune system? Wear protective clothing? And, reconsider how practical it is in some cultures to honor the hottest time of the day with a siesta in respecting nature—thereby sensibly dividing work and play with resting periods?

The foyer of Nidah Spa in the Eldorado Hotel, Santa Fe, New Mexico, pays homage to its namesake, "el dorado" or city of gold, with a stunning gold and copper fresco.

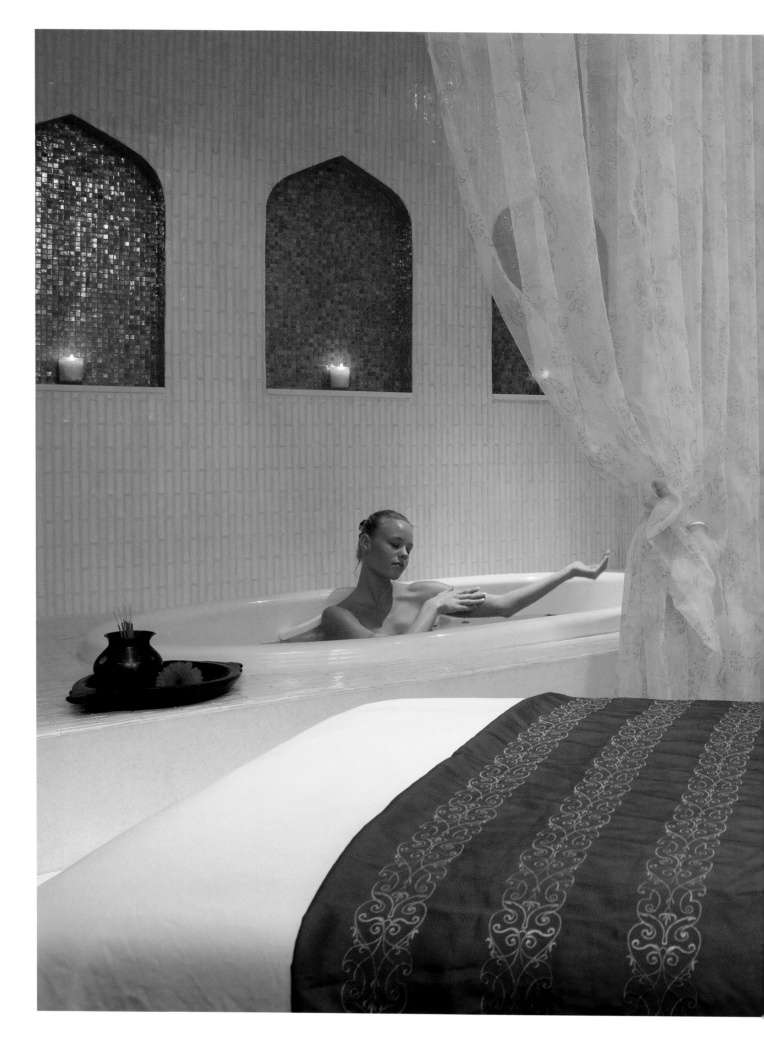

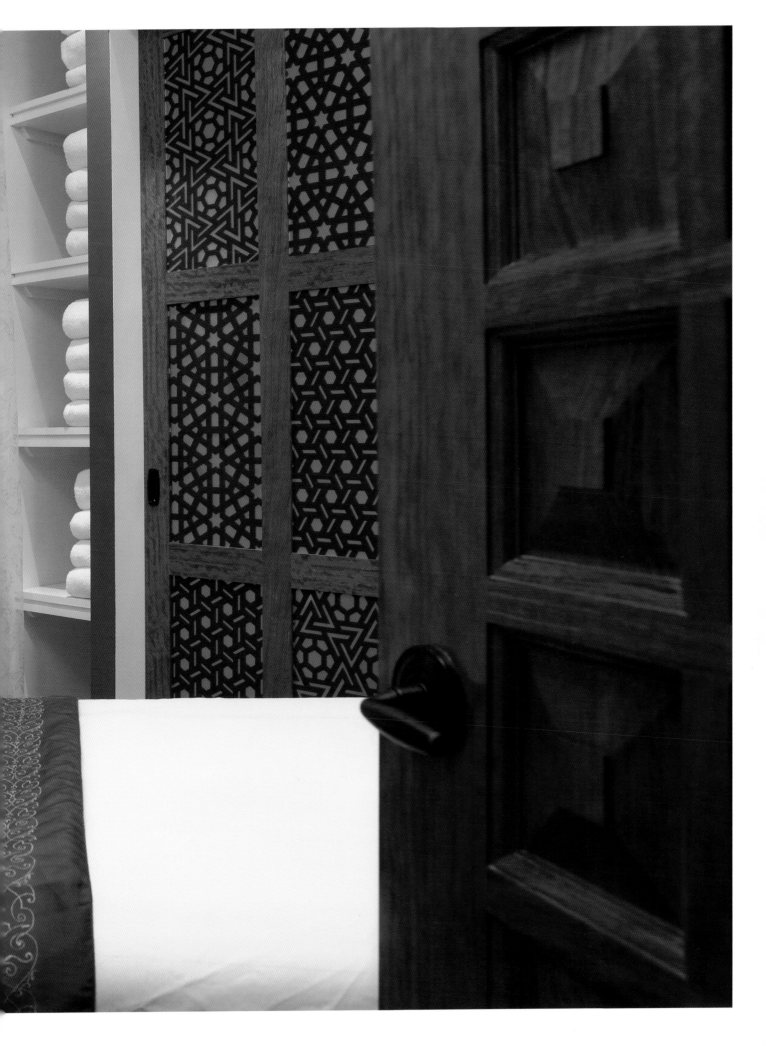

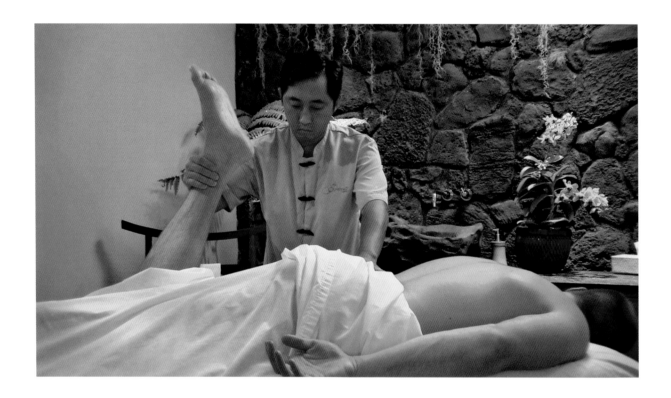

growing under the skin. To avoid them, she advises exfoliating regularly too.

"You can exfoliate with a gentle 'physical' exfoliant containing grains that buff and polish away dead skin cells, or you can also exfoliate with an 'active' exfoliant such as a cream containing alpha hydroxy acid that easily dissolves dead skin cells to reveal smoother, even-toned, and fresher-looking skin. Try applying a toner with salicylic acid directly onto the troublesome area after shaving, and keep applying it for a few days to help prevent new ingrown hairs from developing," Miller advises.

Nicole Morris, spa director at The Westin at Times Square in New York City, says, "To prevent ingrown hair, it is always best to cleanse and apply a warm towel to the face prior to shaving. Use a new blade and rinse the blade after each stroke. Applying an aftershave containing salicylic acid can prevent ingrown hairs too. Remember to find products that are suited for your skin type, and make time for your daily skin-care regimen."

It helps if a spa is adjacent to the gym, which is the case at this Westin, where Morris finds two out of five spa guests are typically male. In Hawaii, Hippo Lipkin sees a ratio of 15 percent male to 85 percent female spa guests visiting Mandara at the Hilton Hawaiian Village in Honolulu; while farther down

previous spread: A Mughal-themed treatment room with its own bathtub at the Chopra Center & Spa at Dream, New York City. (Courtesy photo)

Full-body massage rebalances energy throughout the body again at SpaOlakino, Honolulu. (Courtesy photo)

facing: A sparkly showerhead revitalizes at Cornelia Day Resort & Spa. (Courtesy photo)

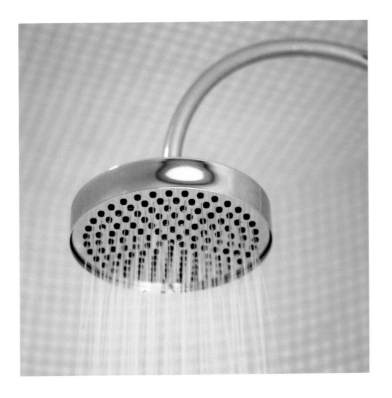

SPA BATHS AT HOME

By Kim Telles, Spa Manager, Tamaya Mist Spa, Hyatt Regency Tamaya Resort & Spa

"While getting an herbal wrap at a spa, please let your service provider know if you are pregnant or if you have high blood pressure, hypothyroidism (thyroid regulates body temperature), or diabetes.

"Spa wraps are difficult to do at home on your own. Instead, I recommend taking your time with spa baths. They are much easier and just as fun and pleasant. Here's a sweet recipe I enjoy at home."

Spa Bath for Home Enjoyment
3 tablespoons rosemary
1 tablespoon lemongrass
3 tablespoons peppermint
1 tablespoon gingerroot

These herbs should be dried, not fresh. They promote mental clarity, stimulate the circulatory system, encourage the body to sweat out toxins, ease muscle aches, and are refreshing and antifungal.

Mix the herbs together. Place in a muslin bag and float in a bath of warm water heated to the desired temperature for your body. Let herbs steep for ten minutes. Then, enjoy both bath and fragrances for as long as you wish.

the road on Kalakaua Avenue, Gary Rohana sees about 30 percent men and 70 percent women frequenting his SpaOlakino.

At Avanyu Spa, "Beauty is so much more than traditional spa treatments today. It's about total health, and the spas that recognize this are the spas that will attract the men," notes director, Dan Mohr.

"In addition to skin care, men want to know more about lifestyles that bring health and beauty. Detoxification, alternative healthcare, and adventure programs are huge draws for men now. Men want to take care of themselves, but they want to have fun while doing it!" Mohr observes.

And if the harried male CEO finds taking time off to jet to exotic spas impossible, he can try relaxing and indulging in the quiet sanctuary of his own home. In 1965, physician Henry G. Bieler advised in his book *Food Is Your Best Medicine*, "About 90 percent of the benefit to the patient taking spa treatment comes from mental relaxation, vacation change and rest, even though the diet (back in the hey day of 'fat farms') is often atrocious at these places. Too, many are very expensive. A week's rest at home, fasting on fruit and vegetable juices and bathing frequently in a tub of warm water to which Epsom salts and Glauber's salts have been added, will accomplish more good with much less drain on the

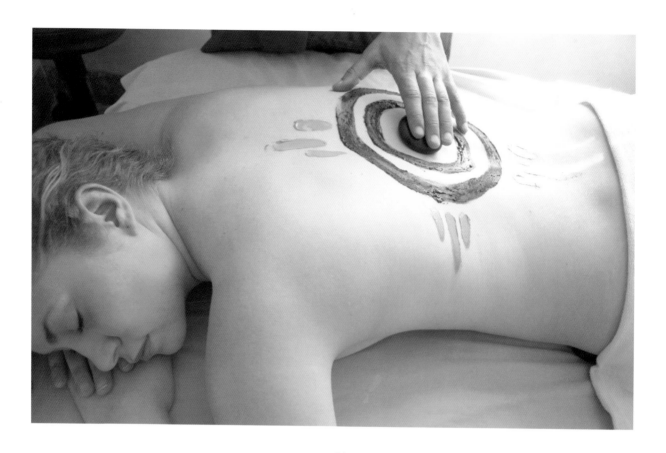

purse, and less strain on the kidneys. This same treatment will also lower an elevated blood pressure."[3]

Everyone interviewed for this book is unequivocal about taking time to care for body, mind, and spirit. And especially in fast-paced urban environments such as New York City, Nicole Morris at The Westin at Times Square emphasizes, "It is essential to maintain a balance in our busy daily schedules. Respecting the proper care of self—from a healthy food intake, exercise program, to adequate sleep—is the foundation for balanced living. Take the time to take care of yourself on a personal level, including detoxifying from the week's activities with a massage or body treatment, to relaxing with a good book; this should be mandatory on everyone's agenda," Morris advises.

Ideally, feeling good about ourselves will inspire "that certain joie de vivre or love of living life to keep learning and growing—for a renewed interest in the world and people around us by doing volunteer or philanthropic work—to radiating an enthusiasm for living life to the fullest," is the earnest wish of Jenean LaRoche, Nob Hill Spa director at The Huntington Hotel in San Francisco.

Prevailing on all four directions to rebalance energy with a Native American treatment at Ojo Caliente Spa. (Courtesy photo)

facing: Setting the ambiance to luxuriate in a relaxing spa bath. (Courtesy photo)

[3] Page 134.

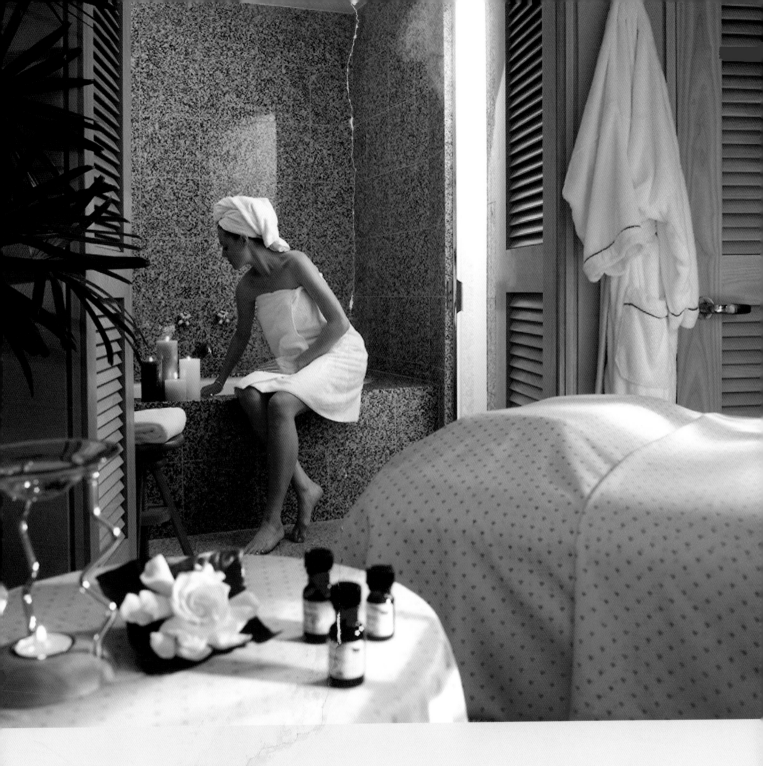

BEING CONSISTENT PAYS

By Andrea Miller, Manager, Golden Door Skin Care

Be consistent with your skin-care regimen. It will confuse the skin if you switch products too often. Find something that works and stick with it. If you are not sure, give it approximately three months to acclimate to your skin. However, if you have an immediate negative reaction, then stop using the product immediately. If you are experiencing challenging breakouts, rashes, or other skin conditions, then please consult with a dermatologist. Note: Consider modifying your regime and/or the products used based on changes in the season, climate, or hormonal fluctuations.

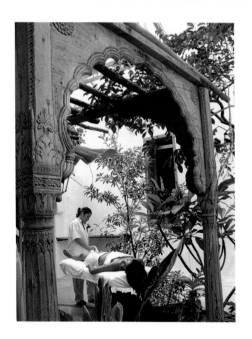

An al fresco courtyard massage invigorates at El Monte Sagrado Living Resort & Spa. (Courtesy photo)

facing: Taking in the fresh air between spa treatments at Avanyu Spa at La Posada de Santa Fe.

Just as important, proper facial skin care is good food for the body:

• It helps strengthen the body's immune system in an area of the anatomy that is constantly exposed to the elements, regardless of the season.

• Because everyone is different and unique, people need to determine from a qualified aesthetician their own skin type, and then use relevant skin-care products.

• Radiant beauty on the face is a reflection of the body's deeper state of health, thus serving as an exterior indicator to rebalance the body's vital energies when needed.

[6] April 13, 2006, by The NPD Group, from an online press release at: http://www.npd.com/press/releases/press_060413.html.

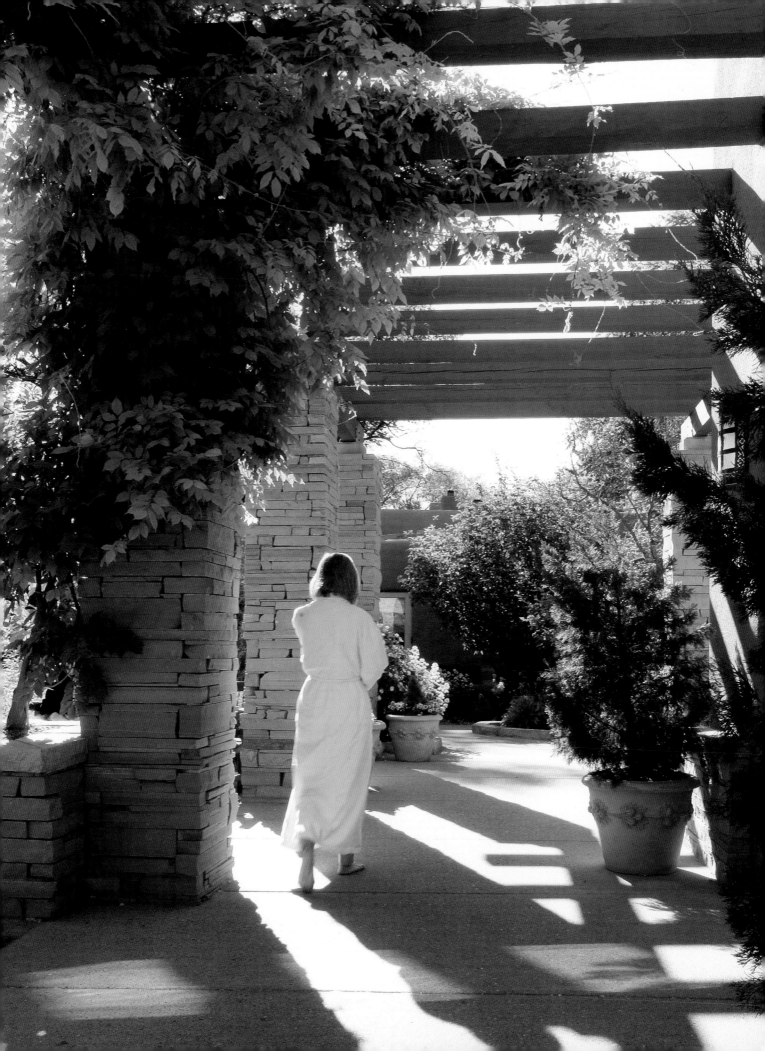

CHAPTER FOUR

BALANCING BODY·MIND·SPIRIT WITH MEDITATION

To live in the beauty

And fragrance of the heart

Is to get younger

By the second.

—Sri Chinmoy, Meditation Master and Powerlifter

Nature's healing elixir is second to none. Just by looking out my east-facing kitchen windows to drink in the morning sky awash in orange and pink against the canvas of an emerging dawn invigorates me immediately—to greet and offer thanks for a new, exciting day ahead, and by so doing, intuitively offer a soulful salutation and meditation to Mother Nature. When I share this simple story in my meditation classes, students immediately identify with similar heartfelt experiences that bring them joy from deep within—be they hiking and enjoying scenic views, or walking barefoot on a smooth, sandy beach.

Meditation is, very simply, being transported to an inner space where mind, body, and spirit are comfortably at ease with one another. Nature's meditation, like music meditation, is spontaneous and joyful in bringing serenity to anyone who is receptive and open to inner quiet. We only need go with the flow of the moment, by allowing ourselves to be transported to other realms of inner harmony—and in doing so, release debilitating stress from our lives.

In my other home reference books,[1] I share how our residence welcomes and rejuvenates us at the end of the day and explore the various ways our homes nurture us. So, too, our garden revitalizes us in similar ways.

A garden "can act as a healing place, where we can substitute

A graceful touch of Bali nurtures the soul at Tonia Prestupa's backyard in Santa Fe, New Mexico.

---

[1] In *Chinese Style: Living in Beauty and Prosperity* and *Japanese Style: Designing with Nature's Beauty*.

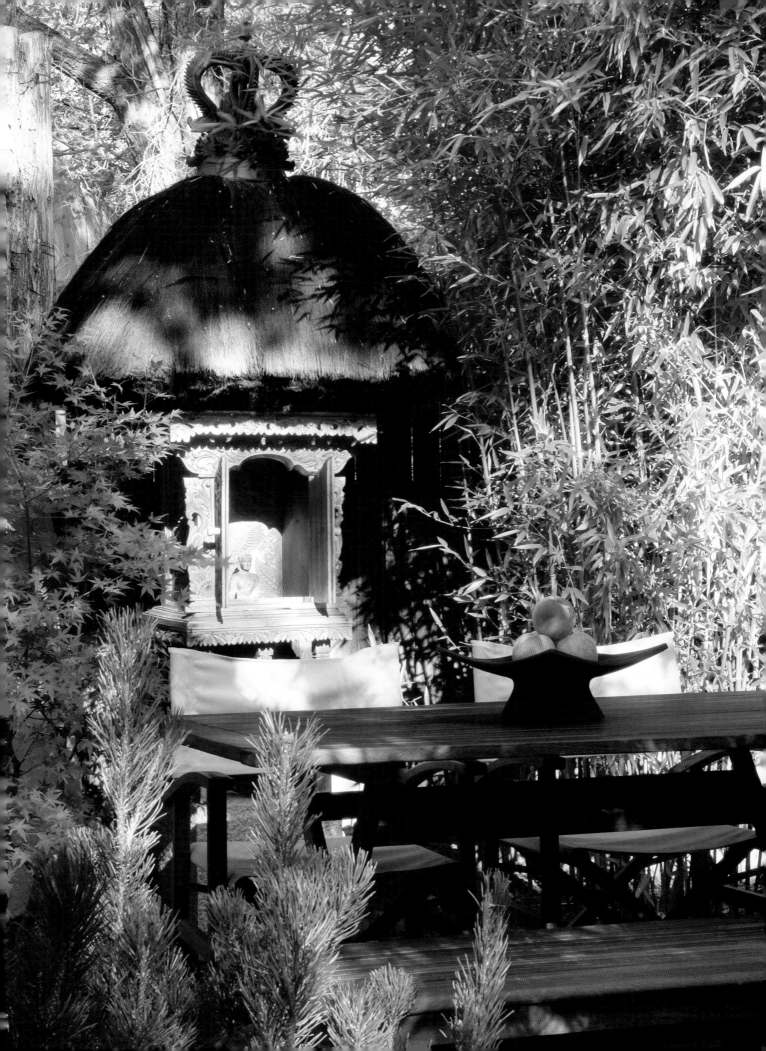

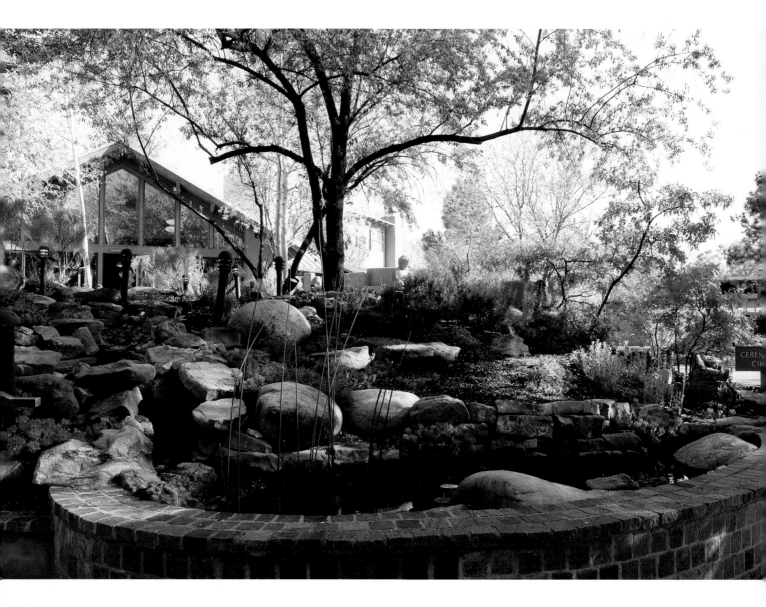

Natural elements lend an earthy grace to Spa Samadhi at Sunrise Springs, Santa Fe.

facing: The coldwater dip refreshes in between takes at Waterfall hot tub and sauna at Ten Thousand Waves Japanese Spa and Retreat, Santa Fe, New Mexico.

soothing images for disturbing ones. . . . In fact, research has shown that hospital patients who can see a tree outside their window heal many times faster than patients without a view of a natural object," writes Julie Messervy in her book, *The Inward Garden* (Little, Brown & Company, 1995). She notes too, "A garden can also be a place of refuge—a sanctuary from the everyday world . . . [while] breathing in its fragrances, all the while contemplating and dreaming. When we lose ourselves in the care of a garden we cherish spending time alone."

Gardening allows you to meditate on nature in a happy, healthy way, rebalancing body-mind-spirit. Messervy continues, "Your garden is the expression of your inner needs, and is not

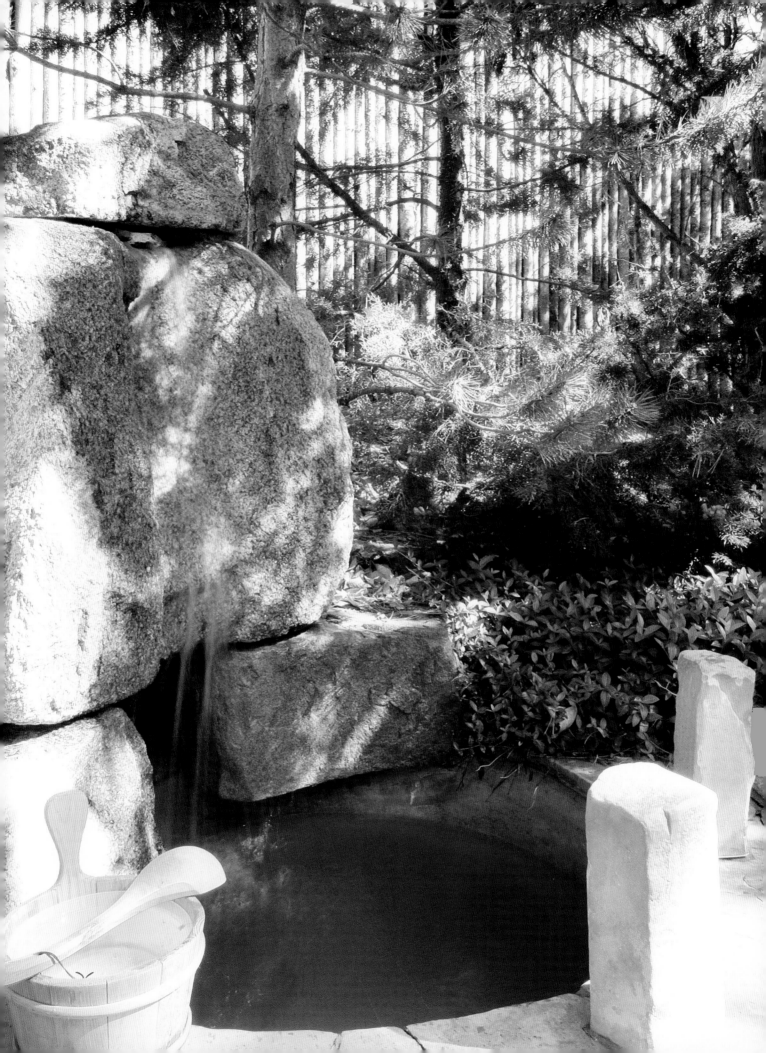

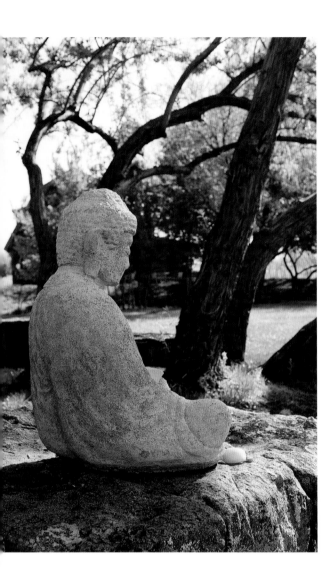

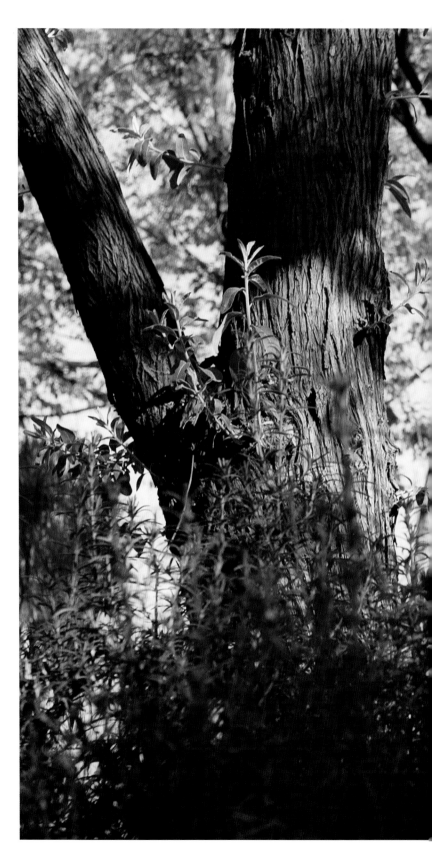

A stone Buddha blesses a peaceful stroll
through the sprawling gardens en route to
Spa Samadhi at Sunrise Springs, Santa Fe.

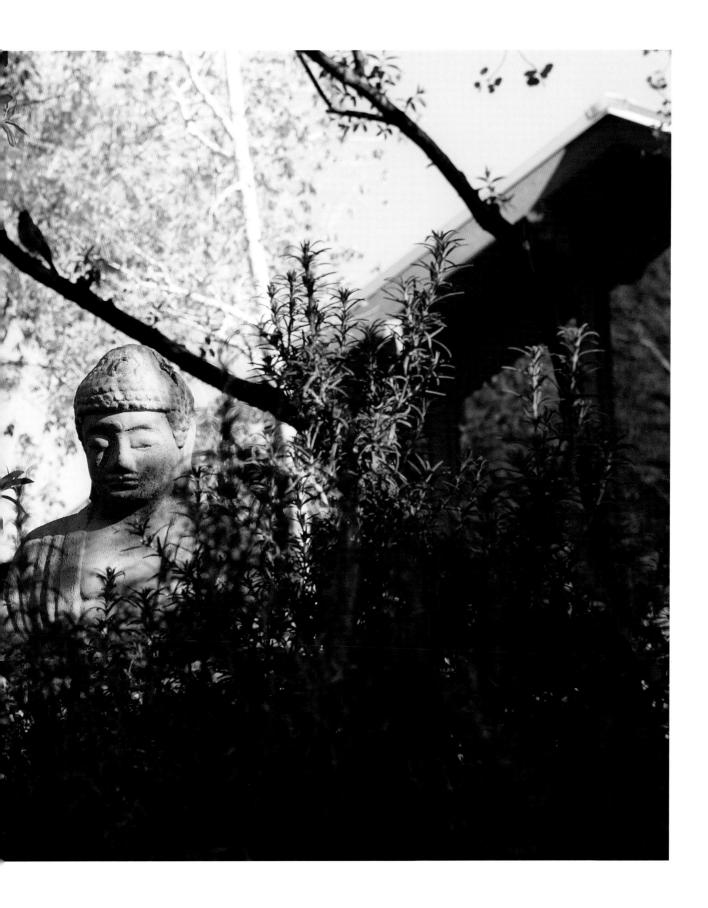

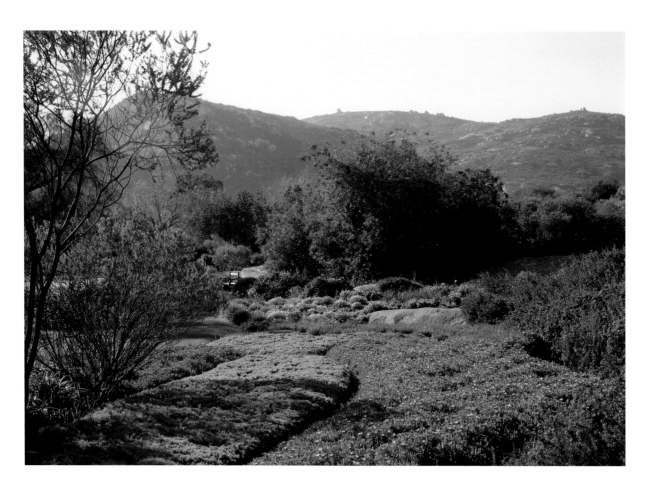

Spring foliage and flora grace the peaceful landscape at Rancho la Puerta. (Courtesy photo)

facing: An invitation to refresh the spirit at Tonia Prestupa's Japanese-style indoor tearoom.

subject to fashion or popular style. . . . In cultivating your garden, you cultivate your soul; in feeding your soul, you can give back more gracefully to this larger garden that we all inhabit."[2] The art of life continues, so that, "After you start gardening you'll find that you can't stop seeing the world as an aesthetic unity,"[3] Messervy observes.

Another passionate gardener and designer who regularly appears on TV, Fran Sorin, writes in *Digging Deep: Unearthing Your Creative Roots through Gardening* (Warner Books, 2004), "Our creative roots make up the very fiber of who we are as individuals, and by unearthing our creative nature, we at the same time unearth our authentic selves. . . . At the end of the day, the reason we create is not for the finished product, but to get to the best parts of ourselves."[4]

What we do with love, sincerity, and intensity (or passion) also necessitates digging deep inwardly to achieve the most satisfying results. Sorin's and Messervy's garden metaphors drive home this point vividly.

[2] Page 20.

[3] Ibid., 201.

[4] Pages xii–xiii.

HOW TO MAKE GOOD TEA

By John Harney, Master Tea Blender, Harney & Sons Fine Teas

A good pot of tea cannot be made from bad tea. Always use quality tea leaves or sachets with larger tea leaves in them. Here are my guidelines:

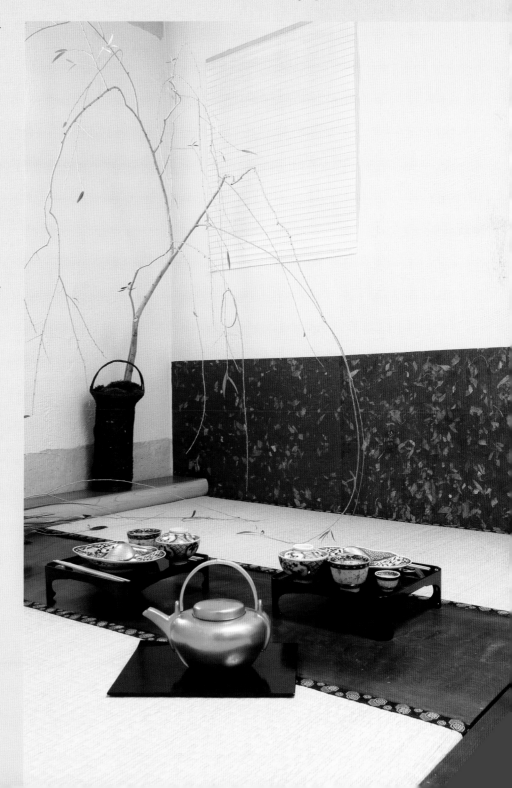

1. Start by using fresh, filtered, or spring water, and a level teaspoon of loose tea for every cup, plus one extra for the pot.

2. Preheat teapot by pouring boiling water into it, to raise the interior temperature to the correct 180 degrees Fahrenheit.

3. Swish the boiling water in the teapot to warm it up; then discard.

4. Next, add tea. Pour boiling water over tea to saturate it for a more flavorful extraction. Adding tea to standing hot water is wrong, as it results in a lower temperature and therefore, poor tea.

5. Steeping times: for black, white, oolong, and herbal teas, steep at least 4–5 minutes; for green tea, use less than boiling water and steep 1–3 minutes. Place the lid on and allow the tea to steep, covered.

6. Strain and pour into a warm teacup. The flavor is enhanced by serving tea in fine bone china or porcelain teacups that results in a luxurious "cuppa," both soothing and satisfying.

7. Black tea may be served with milk and sugar.

GETTING STARTED IN MEDITATION AT HOME OR IN THE OFFICE

1. Clear out and clean up an area—by your bed, a corner cranny, or space on your desk—and spread a clean light-colored fabric over it.

2. Place an object or two that inspires you on the clean fabric: a floral arrangement; a photograph of Christ, Buddha, or whoever inspires you, including your children, of a sunset, or a soft, impressionist painting by Monet; and a candle, if you like. Incense helps purify the air and the overall ambiance.

3. Sit up straight, facing your portable meditation shrine.

4. Gently loosen up your neck and shoulder muscles by turning your head clockwise and then counterclockwise a few times.

5. Feel tension dribbling off and trickling down your arms as you loosen them.

6. Half-close your eyes as in a lion's meditation, with one

continued

Welcoming Nature's beauty into our lives can take other forms that are meditative, healing, and fulfilling, as well. Have you noticed how serene a quilter's living room feels? How tranquil a potter's studio is, and as earthy as it smells? Do you enjoy the uplifting aromas of freshly baked bread and chocolate chip cookies as they waft through your house? Taking time to enjoy a cup of freshly brewed tea, while being reinvigorated with subtle aromas that tingle the nostrils and heighten the senses?

In a nutshell, we can be as creatively meditative as we want to be, in whatever mode we enjoy—gardening, cooking, cleaning, reading, running—to feel totally happy, at peace, secure, and fulfilled with our lives. This is the simple secret of inviting meditation into our daily activities, if only for a few moments daily—to be cleansed and purified by staying in the heart, and engaging in activities that rebalance us with new joy and energy.

"To rebalance the mind-body-spirit disharmony, I suggest learning to meditate to invite peaceful energy into a person's consciousness. We're big on mindfulness here at Miraval Resort. We advocate developing awareness in all actions—eating, making decisions, relaxing, and living life with a deeper satisfaction."

—Donald Kimon Lightner, Licensed Acupuncturist, Miraval Resort & Spa, Tucson, Arizona

facing: Nature meditation is easy to enjoy in a serene setting.

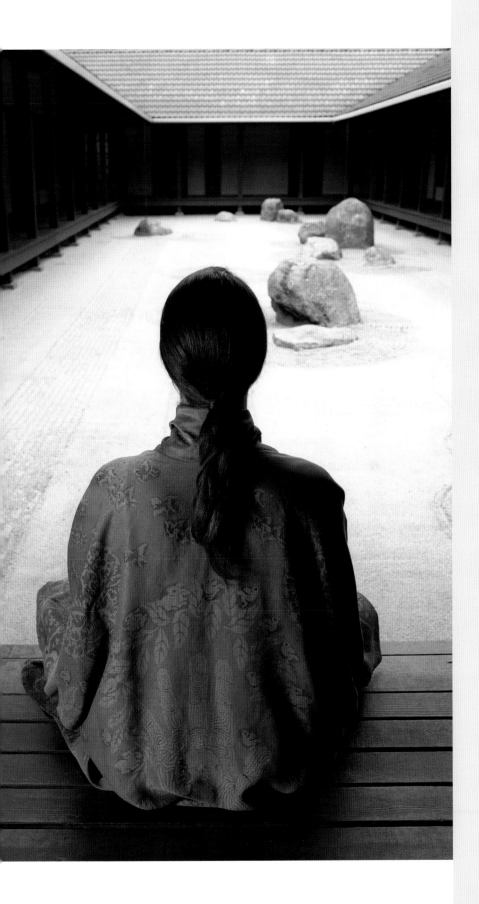

foot on the inner plane and the other on the outer—ready to tune in to Nature's offerings.

7. Have your hands resting on your lap, Tweedledee and Tweedledum, where they're gently reposed and not distracting you.

8. Then, consciously breathe in slowly, and deeply. Start counting at your own pace. The key here is to consciously **breathe deeply**, and to expel all old energy.

9. Inhale as you count—one, two—for peaceful energy to enter into your body; hold—three, four—as you feel this new energy expanding into every pore of your being; and then gently exhale—five, six—as you release restless energy back to the universe.

10. Continue repeating until you feel these new waves of energy purifying your whole being so that you're inhaling *and* exhaling peaceful energy, as well.

11. Gently allow your meditation vessel to be filled with peaceful energy and quiet happiness.

continued

12. As all good thoughts are for sharing and enjoying, next imagine a dear one ready and grateful to receive your goodwill and blessings.

13. Begin sending peaceful messages to this person with your sincere intentions. Do not worry about how receptive this person is. Chances are, because of your soul's connection, this person's soul is aware of your messages of goodwill. (This is one of the first meditation exercises we attempt in class. Many students later recount how their friend or spouse had actually been feeling or thinking about them while we were doing this exercise.)

14. Be sure to include quiet time after each session, to better assimilate your experiences, before reentering into the hustle and bustle of life.

15. Note: If you feel some hunger pangs before starting to meditate, it's okay to eat a piece of fruit and/or drink water before beginning; but a full meal before meditating is not advisable.

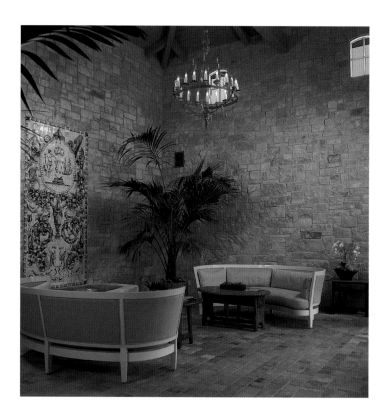

Q: *How do I know I'm meditating correctly?*

Sri Chinmoy: If you are meditating properly, you will feel spontaneous inner joy and peace within and without. But if you feel mental tension or disturbance, then the kind of meditation that you are doing is not meant for you. If you have a good meditation, you will have a good feeling for the world. You will see the world in a loving way in spite of its teeming imperfections . . . [and] also if you have a dynamic feeling right after your meditation.

Please do not be disturbed if you cannot meditate well in the beginning. Even in the outer life, God alone knows how many years one must practice in order to become very good at something. —*Wings of Joy*, pages 37–38

It is easy to lose oneself in Cal-a-Vie's huge fitness center foyer with its blue-white tiled fresco, limestone walls, and antique terracotta floors—and to forget fitness activities down the hall. (Courtesy photo)

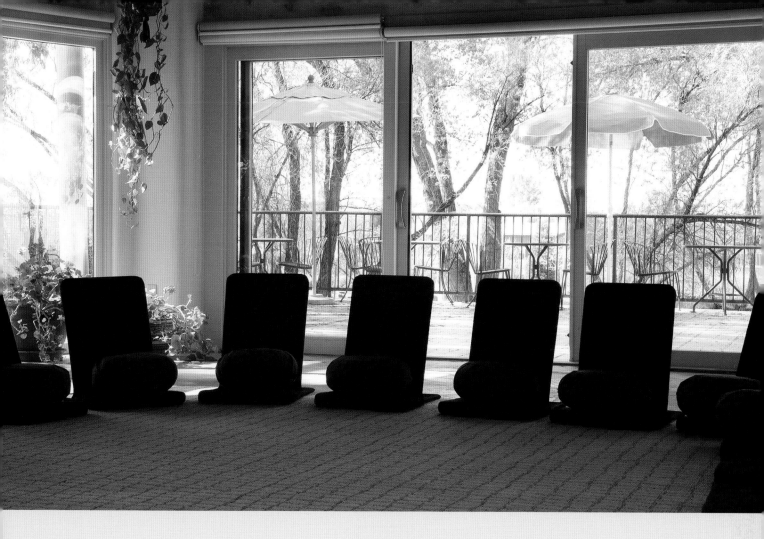

PRACTICAL APPLICATIONS OF A
BREATHING MEDITATION TECHNIQUE

This is a simple pocket breathing meditation you can pull out to refresh sagging spirits, whenever you need new energy and inspiration to continue with the day's activities.

You can try other variations of this exercise. Whenever you need to refuel your body-mind-spirit with a desired positive attribute, simply and effectively expel the obverse negative. For example, if you need joy, breathe out resentment, until you feel forgiveness for yourself, the other person, or situation; thereby allowing you to freely breathe in and out, moments of joyful living again.

Another fun variation is the "3 o'clock meditation twinkie." Instead of reaching for outer calories that provide momentary gratification, enjoy instead increased energy (minus the calories) by:

• closing your eyes momentarily,

• breathing in deeply, power; consciously feel this expansive surge of
  pure, powerful energy revitalizing your body-mind consciousness, and

• blessing your entire being with renewed vigor as your toes tingle, and
  warm waves of love and appreciation begin to gently stir in your heart.

**The meditation room at
Sunrise Springs, Santa Fe,
invites in light and nature.**

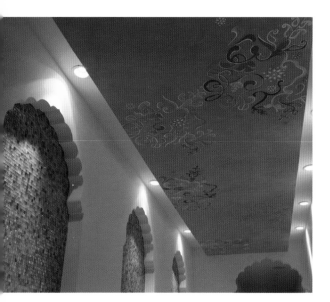

Frescoed ceilings and Mughal motifs provide quiet inspiration at the Chopra Center & Spa at Dream, New York City. (Courtesy photo)

facing: A waiting room-in-the-round at the Chopra Center & Spa at Dream, New York City. (Courtesy photo)

Sri Chinmoy: We say somebody is practical when he does the right thing at the right moment, so that his outer life runs smoothly. But no matter how clever we are, how conscious we are, at times we are at a loss in the outer life. We do not know what to say or do. Or, despite our saying and doing the right thing, everything goes wrong.

Why does this happen? It happens because our outer capacity is always bound by our inner awareness. If we are practical in the inner life, that is to say, if we pray and meditate, then we will increase our inner awareness. When we have inner awareness, we have free access to infinite truth and everlasting joy, and we are able to control our outer life.

We always grow from within, not from without. It is from the seed under the ground that a plant grows, not vice versa. The inner life constantly carries the message of Truth and God. This inner Truth is the seed.

No matter how many hours we work, or talk, or do anything in the outer world, we will not approach the Truth. But if we meditate first, and afterward act and speak, then we are doing the practical thing. —*Wings of Joy*, pages 38–39

GUIDELINES TO KNOW MEDITATION IS WORKING

Meditation is the normal birthright of every individual. Learning to meditate is like getting reacquainted with an old friend again; it's easy to reconnect with it. Your inner pilot is your best guide—so go with your intuitive responses, and learn to listen from within to your innermost self, to your own Soul's Light. Three stellar guidelines that meditation is working are

- When you feel a deep sense of well-being from the very depths of your heart.

- When your mind is at peace, and not contradicting nor dictating your heartfelt feelings welling up from within.

- When you relax and entrust your inner pilot to instinctively guide you to breathe deeply, have faith in your meditation taking you on to new adventures, and let go of expectations of how meditation ought to proceed.

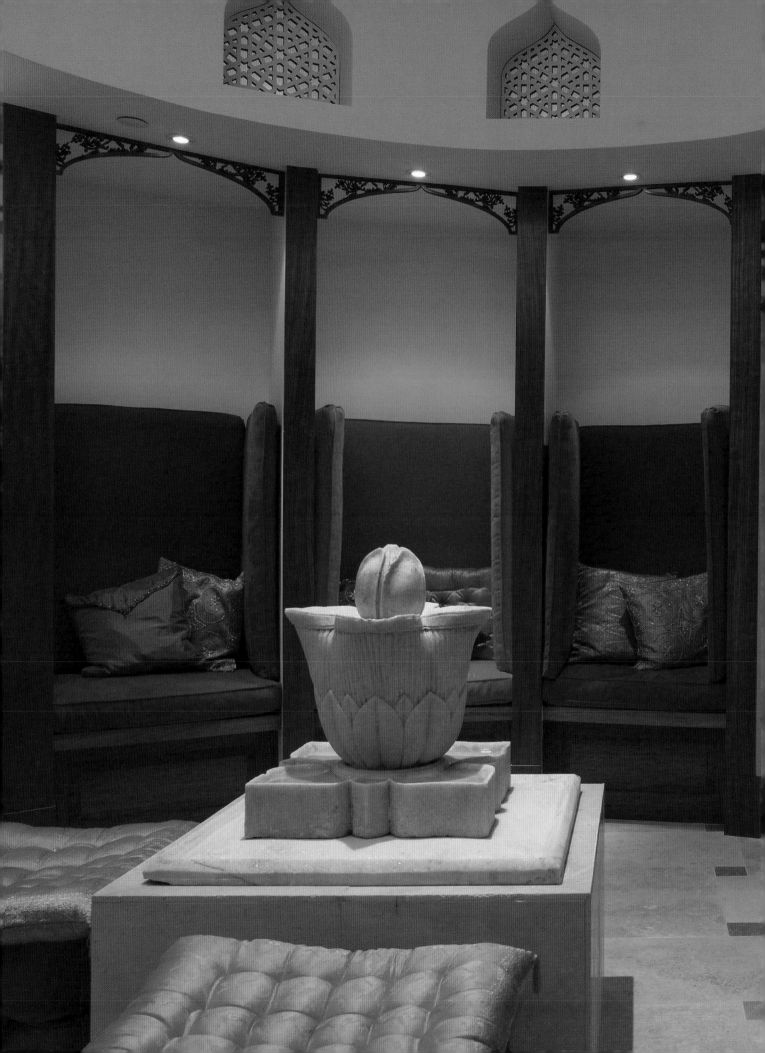

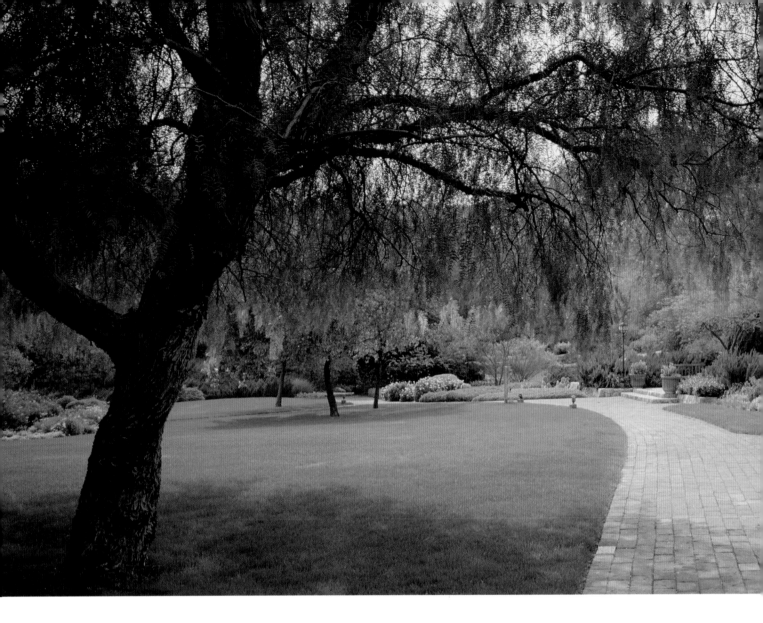

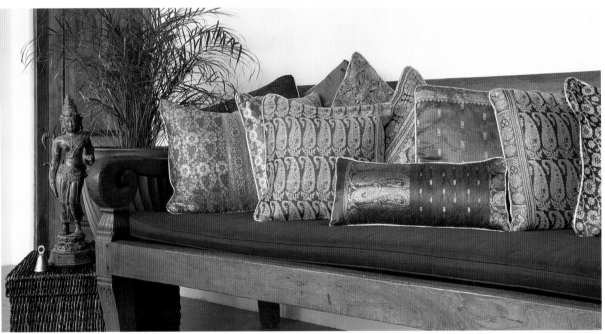

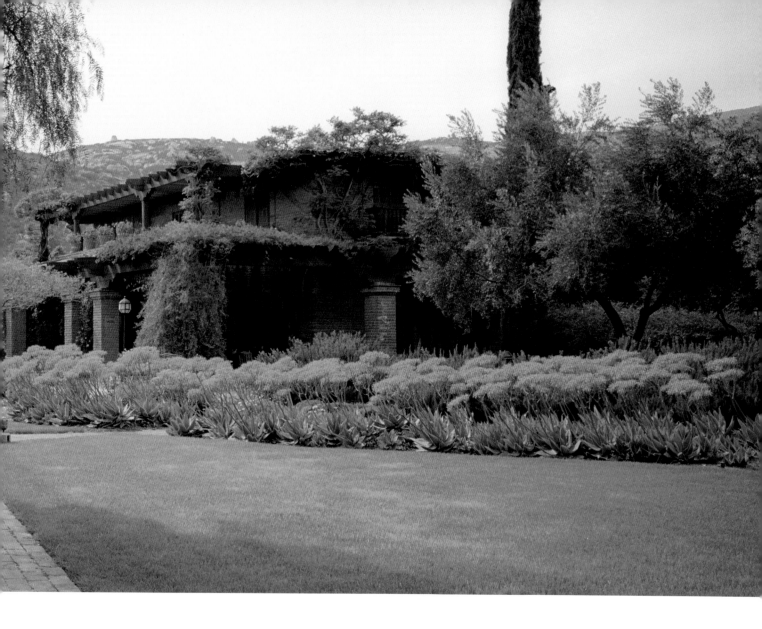

Q: *What is the difference between meditating in the heart and meditating in the mind?*

Sri Chinmoy: The heart is the mother—the mother of love, affection, light, patience, and forgiveness. Once we truly feel that the heart embodies all these divine qualities then we will be able to bring the confidence of the heart into the mind very swiftly, effectively, and fruitfully.

We must feel that the mind is a restless child, without wisdom and maturity, and that the heart is the mother who embodies all divine qualities. Naturally, whatever the mother has, the child can claim because the mother is ready to give whatever she has to the child. So when we think of the heart, we think of the Divine Mother, whose boundless qualities enter into the child while she instructs him. Then, automatically, like a river flowing, the heart's confidence enters into the mind. —*Wings of Joy*, page 105

Well-tended gardens exude peaceful energy for spa guests to enjoy the sanctuary of Rancho la Puerta. (Courtesy photo)

left: A colorful profusion of silk-covered cushions transports guests at Absolute Nirvana Spa in Santa Fe, New Mexico, to the tropics on this Indonesian teak settee.

THREE "TIMELY" MEDITATION QUESTIONS

- *How long should I meditate?* A few minutes to begin with, and gradually building up to fifteen to twenty minutes at a stretch. The key here is to focus on your meditation without being distracted by thoughts and anxieties.

- *When should I meditate?* As morning shows the day, so too, your meditation paves the day ahead with new aspirations to living life purposefully and with a deeper sense of satisfaction. Before lunch and bedtime are also helpful to empty your consciousness of the day's accumulated emotional debris.

- *How often should I meditate?* As often as your inner pilot beckons—that is, whenever you feel an intuitive need to tune-up and rebalance your life by becoming more calm and focused.

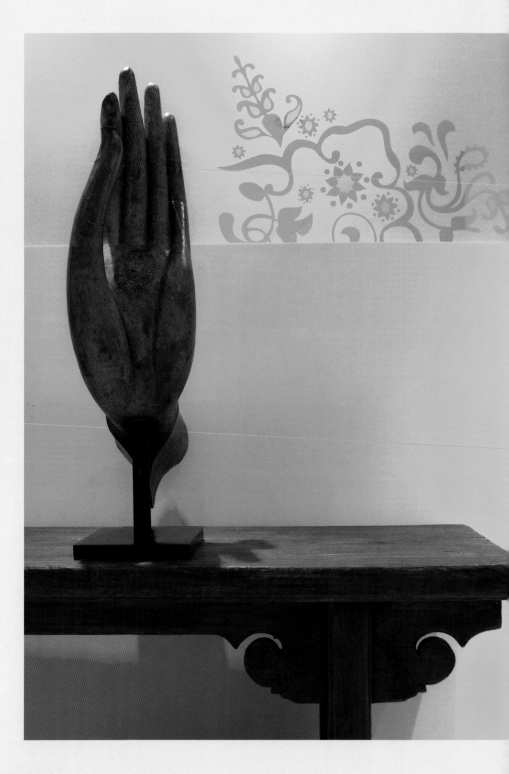

A symbolic meeting of Mughal and Chinese aesthetics at the Chopra Center & Spa at Dream, New York City. (Courtesy photo)

facing: A serene, plush corner offers simple sustenance at Cornelia Day Resort & Spa. (Courtesy photo)

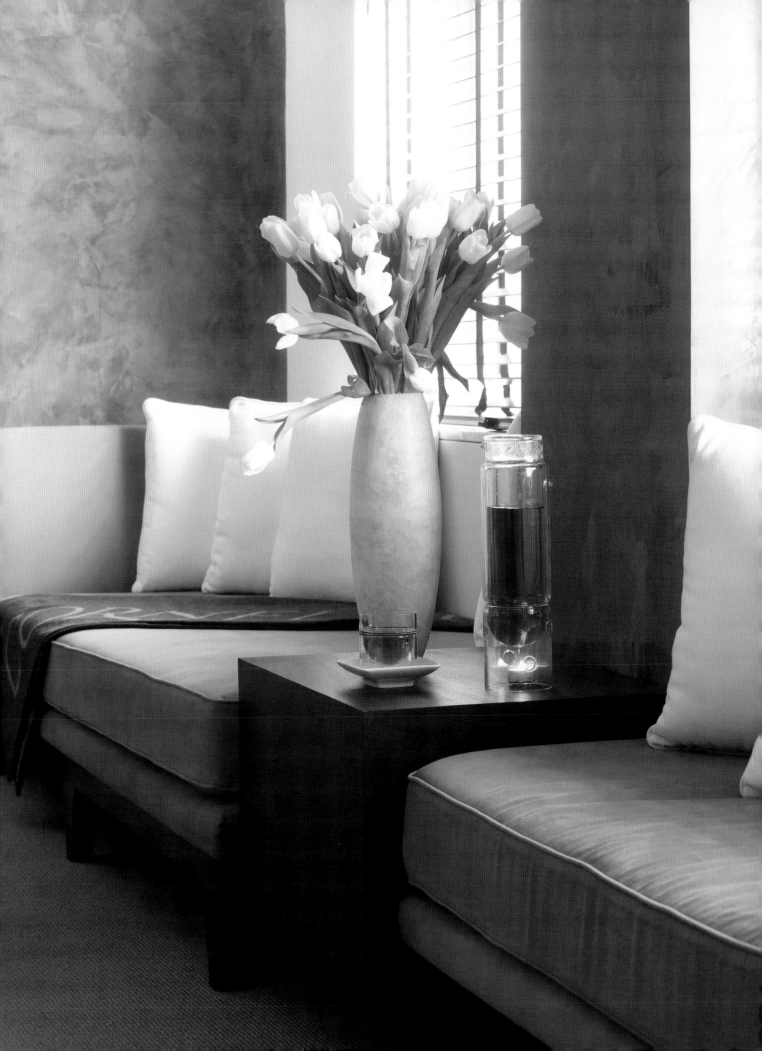

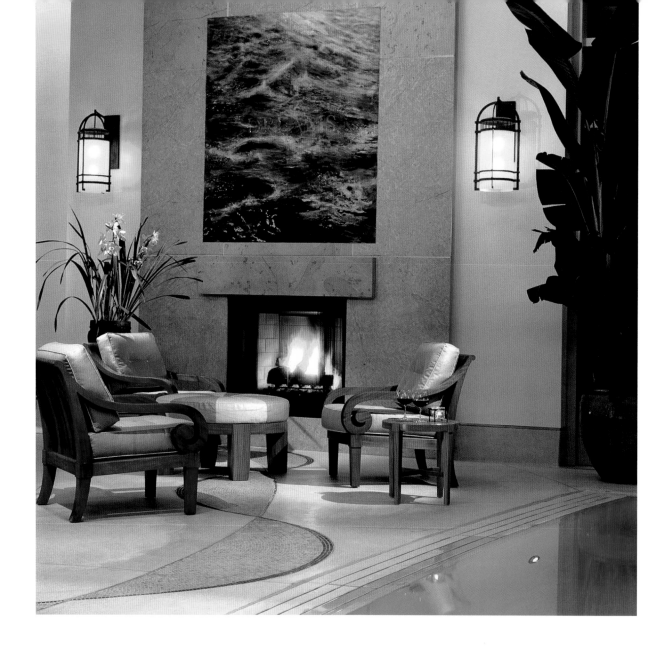

Fireplace splendor by Nob Hill Spa's
indoor pool at The Huntington Hotel in
San Francisco. (Courtesy photo)

facing: Indoor cabanas by the pool at the
Palm Springs Parker Meridien Spa in
California. (Courtesy photo)

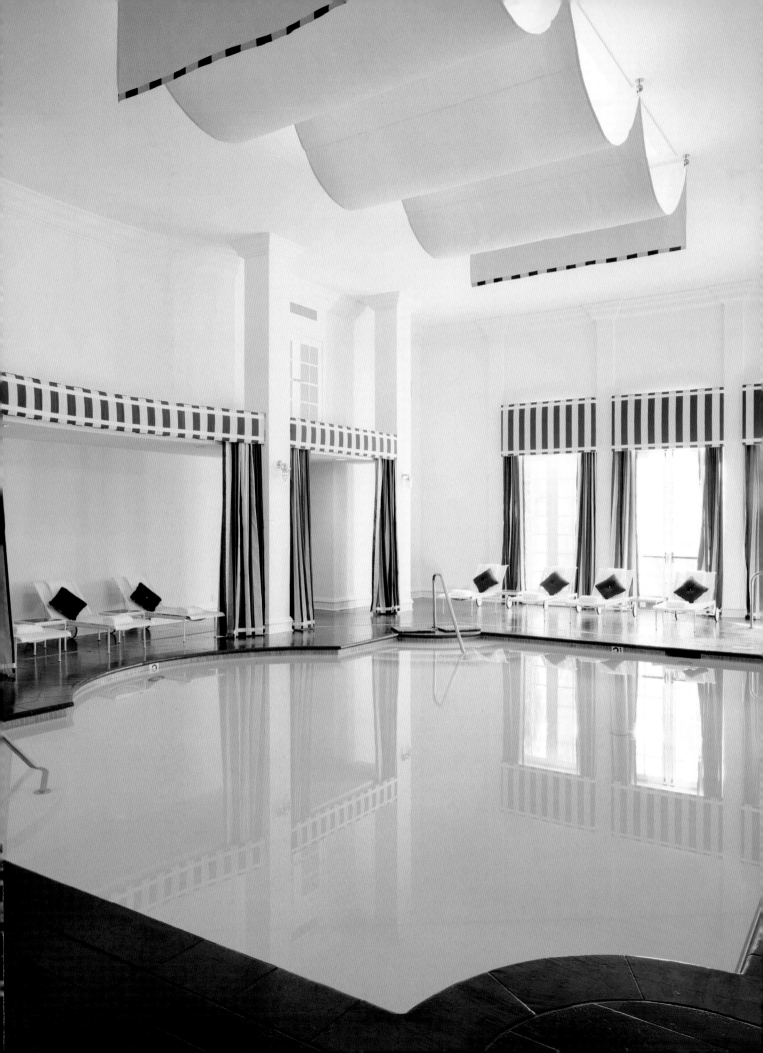

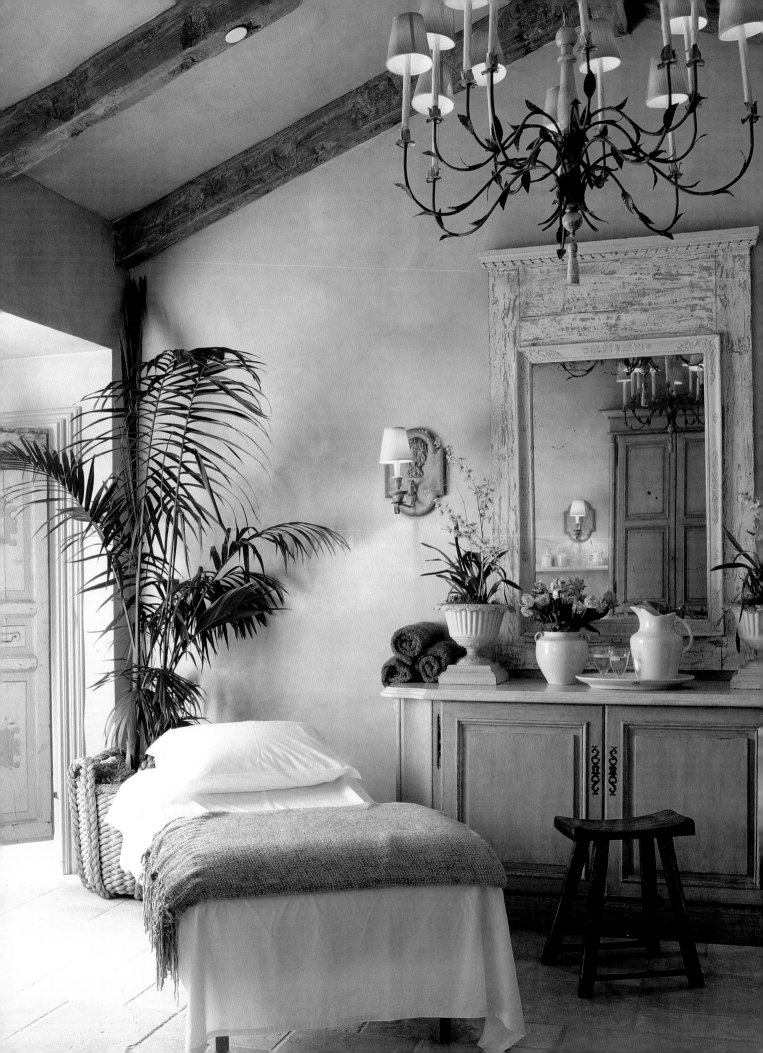

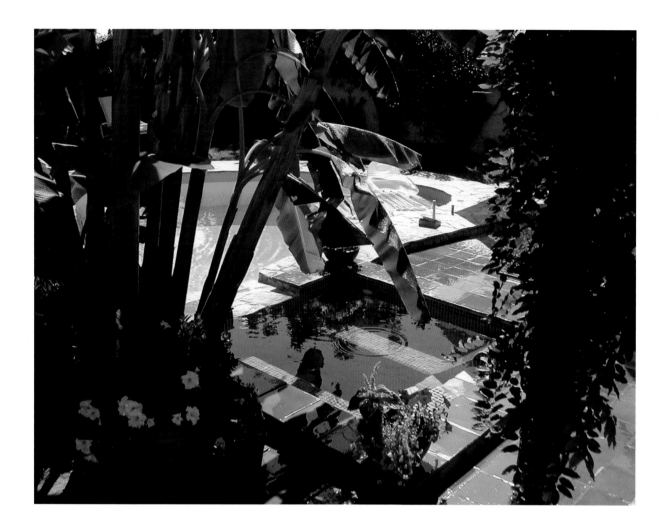

THREE TIPS FOR
GETTING READY TO MEDITATE

- Unplug your home/office phone and turn off your cell phone.

- Loosen your clothing—unbutton, unbuckle, and kick off your shoes.

- Sit up straight, naturally. Sitting on a chair to meditate is good, but try not to use the back splat for support as a laid-back posture may encourage daydreaming and drowsiness.

Siesta Spa's minipool has built-in massage jets to unknot tired muscles. (Courtesy photo)

facing: A treatment room at Cal-a-Vie is decorated with French-style fixtures and furnishings. The antique French tole chandelier is from the home of owners John and Terri Havens. (Courtesy photo)

CHAPTER FIVE

ATTAINING PHYSICAL AND EMOTIONAL FITNESS

Physical exercise is an inner massage. Like cutaneous massage, it works the muscles to relieve tension, tone the skin, improve circulation, and stimulate lymphatic flow. As such, it is a vital part of any health and beauty routine.

—Pratima Raichur, ND, Author of *Absolute Beauty* (HarperPerennial, 1997), founder of Pratima Skin Care Salon, and creator of Bindi, Tej, and Ojas Ayurvedic beauty lines

Attaining a balanced and powerful state of physical fitness is not only the athlete's goal, but is aspired to by many, as well. We are living longer life spans today. But ultimately, it is the quality of life that matters—to live life filled with inspirations that satisfy from deep within, enjoying optimal health and a continuous sense of well-being.

How Physical Fitness Energizes—with Oxygen

As much of an oxymoron as it sounds, dynamic energy as a result of physical movement and exercise does fuel peaceful energy, which in turn fosters creativity and moments of transcendent awareness and bliss for artists, and those so in tune with themselves too.

This is how long-distance runner and acclaimed wood-turning sculptor David Nittmann is, by his own account, "creatively nurtured by running meditation." Nittmann runs on trails 9,000 feet above sea level around Boulder, Colorado, where he lives; he celebrated his sixty-second birthday running 26.2 miles, the equivalent of a marathon.

Hailed by collectors for his trailblazing wood artistry, Nittmann turns, burns, and designs museum-quality pieces that resemble platters and bowls woven by Native American Pueblo artisans. Except, Nittmann's intricate "weaving" is executed via

Instructor Steve revives body energy with fluid movements of tai chi at Sunrise Springs, Santa Fe.

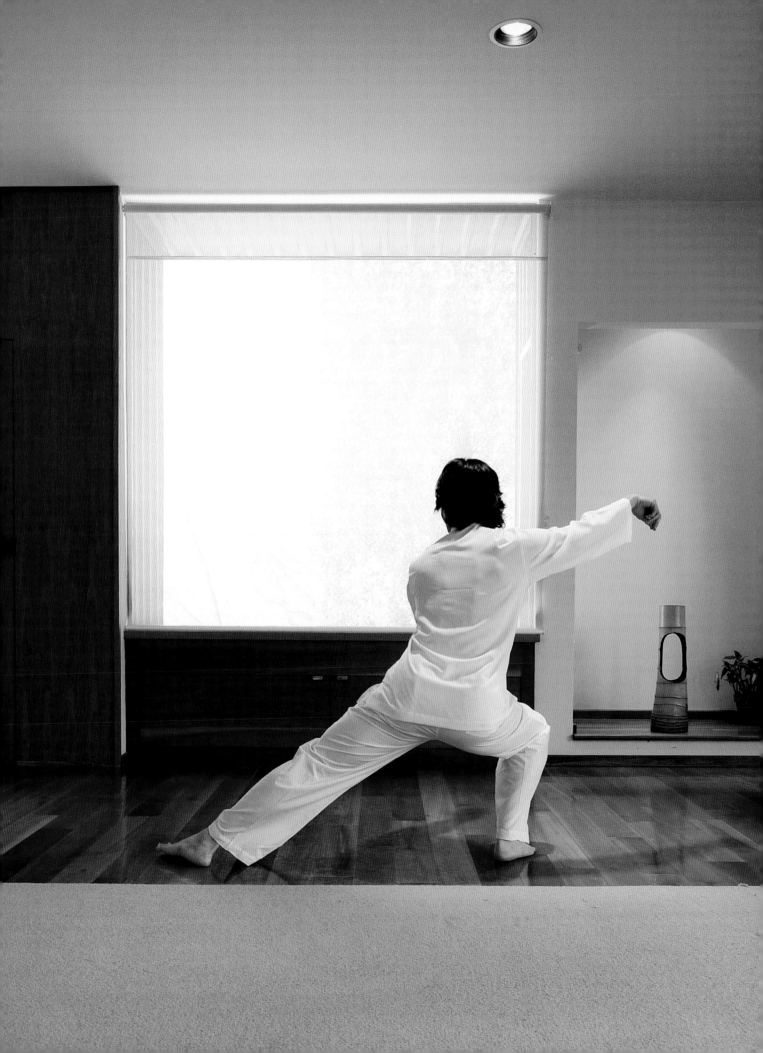

"Exercise promotes oxygen and blood circulation. Have you noticed how runners have the softest skin on their legs?" asks Suk Mancinelli, Spa Manager, Four Seasons Hotel, New York City. While running helps the body sweat and therefore aids in ridding the body of toxins, Mancinelli also suggests:

- Try to be in bed by 10 p.m., to better assist the skin, your body's largest organ, to detoxify, and start healing from the day's activities.
- Enlist the help of your aesthetician to select relevant products for your skin's changing conditions, as it varies according to season and the climate you're in.
- Try to detoxify internally too, in tune with seasonal changes.
- Eat lots of fresh vegetables and fruits to stay alkaline.
- Drink lots of water—at least 2.5 liters (about 5 pints) daily.
- Don't forget to rest up and get enough sleep.
- Be happy, and stay away from toxic stress!

Exercise balls at New York City's Gravity Fitness and Spa at the Parker Meridien. (Courtesy photo)

facing: The journey is worth the destination at Rancho la Puerta's sprawling estate. (Courtesy photo)

lathe and pigmented inks that look incredibly like hand-woven, polychromed basketry.

Another long-distance runner who has completed 100 marathons, as well as a 700-mile ultra-marathon to her credit, finds that fitness and strength through running is her secret to true inner and outer beauty. Sulochana Kallai was an aesthetician with the flagship Saks Beauty Salon on Fifth Avenue in New York City for twenty years.

She opened her beauty salon in July 1984, God's Beauty Skin Care, in Jamaica, New York. In fact, the name for her salon came to her while she was running, she says. In her seventies, Kallai (who was born in Hungary in 1930) continues offering facials, pedicures, and manicures, while keeping up her beauty regimen, which includes daily two-mile runs and meditations of varying lengths throughout the day.

The whole idea is "to get fresh air into your lungs and body," advises this aesthetician, "because fresh air smelling of nature's sweet and earthy fragrances, whether in summer or winter, naturally reinvigorates you."

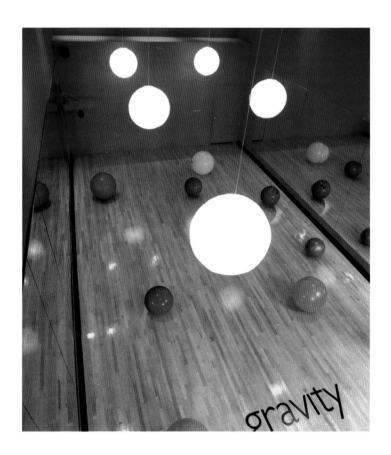

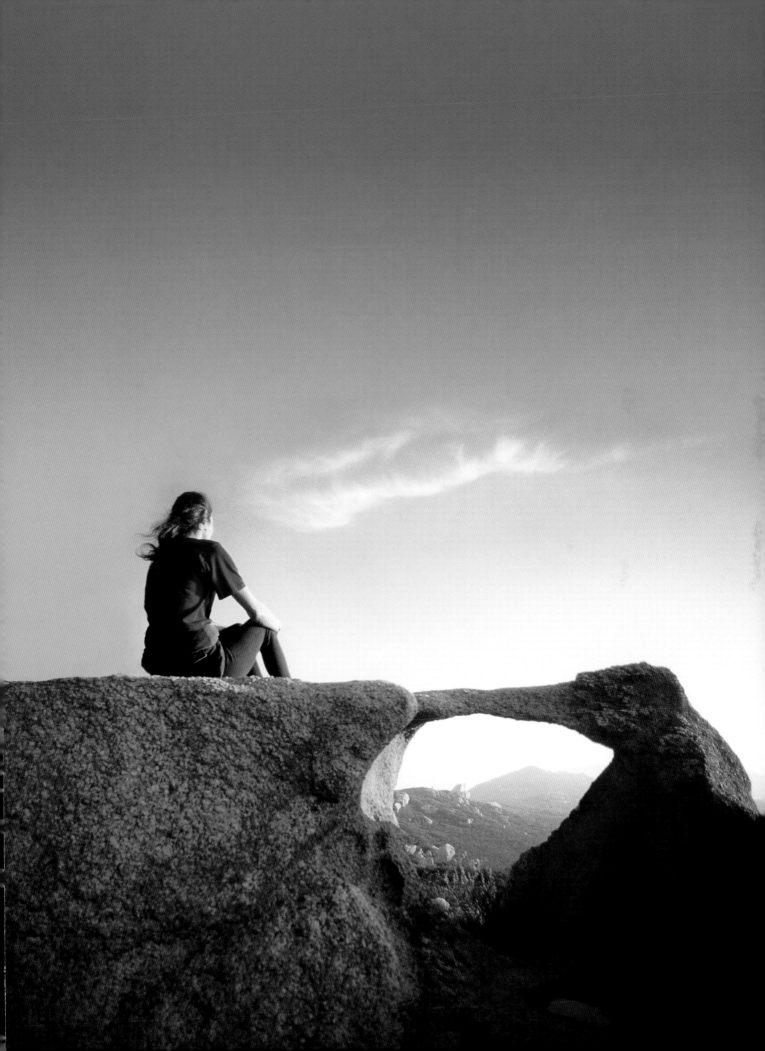

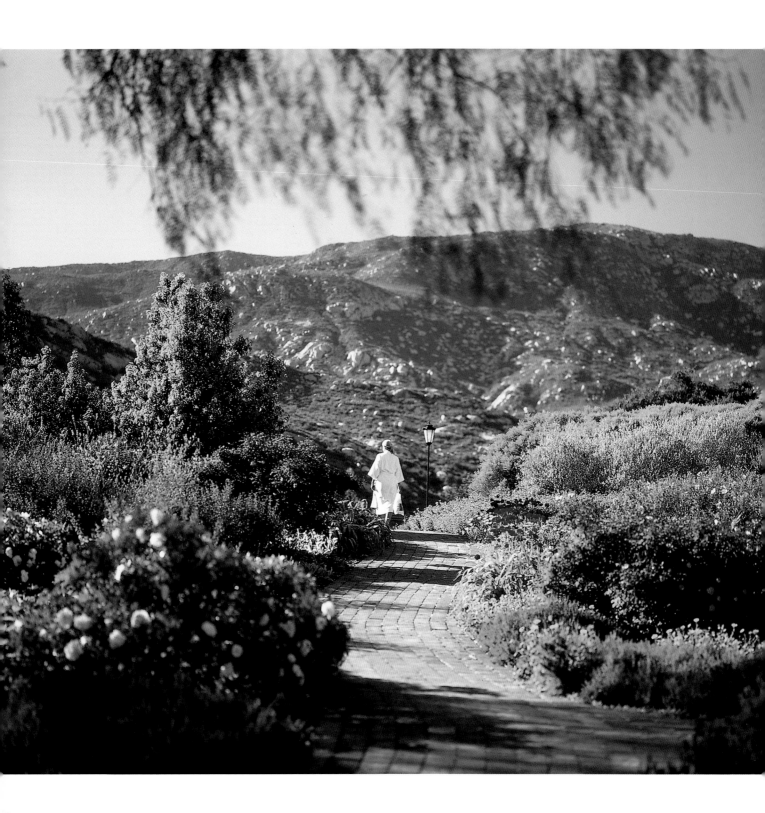

Kallai cautions though, "Trying to get your exercise on a treadmill indoors is *not* the same as exercising outdoors where your lungs get the full benefit of fresh oxygen because our body cells are nourished and rejuvenated by the big 'O'—oxygen!" she proclaims.

Also, pounding on a mechanical treadmill is very different from running on the ground that gives naturally, as each footstep falls on the ground. Kallai is convinced of this from decades of observing her body in motion, and in working with a beauty regimen that blesses her with all-around fitness—physically, emotionally, and spiritually.

This aesthetician is also averse to acquiring artificial tans with solar beds and chemical ointments. "The unnatural rays and chemicals get absorbed into your body; they are so harmful. How can you remain healthy over the long haul?" Kallai asks. It's a perplexing irony to her, "when, so many people pay big bucks to look healthy with unnatural ways of tanning."

"The real beauty," Kallai advocates, "is from within. Outer beauty is skin deep. But inner beauty is everything. Why? Because everything comes from God! Running helps me get closer to my inner pilot, and I'm blessed with all kinds of miraculous experiences," Kallai enthuses. And an emphatic statement in sharing her life's enriching experiences through God's Beauty is her skin-care salon.

The Transformational Power of Water

Lest we forget, water is another powerful, elemental force of nature that energizes and transforms our consciousness, but ever so subtly. Continuously flowing along its course (unless caught in

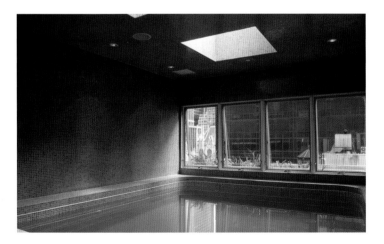

The True Power of Water (Beyond Words, 2005) is a fascinating and credible read by Japanese physician and researcher Dr. Masaru Emoto. Dr. Emoto's research reveals how:

- Water heals, by reflecting our dispositions. With positive feelings of love, water molecules respond with beautiful, complex shapes, while negative thoughts disintegrate water molecules into misshapen forms.

- Given the larger fabric of cosmic interactions, water transforms the nature of energy for positive uses. Sincere intentions and prayers can resound in subtle, healing, vibratory effects.

Encouraged by Shintoism's emphasis on purification with water rituals and cleansing baths, Japanese culture has always respected cleanliness. *The Japanese Bath* by Bruce Smith and Yoshiko Yamamoto (Gibbs Smith, 2001) is an informative guide to enjoying the way of *furo* (Japanese bath)—that heals and transforms in an aqueous manner, social and family relationships at the end of the day. Taking time to soak away stress is, indeed, a graceful way to exit the day.

facing: Leisurely strolls bestow an uncommon serenity for spa guests at Rancho la Puerta. (Courtesy photo)

The first *watsu* pool in New York City at Cornelia Day Resort & Spa. (Courtesy photo)

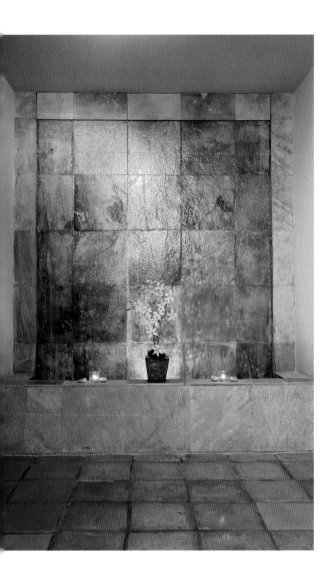

Spa Samadhi's foyer at Sunrise Springs, Santa Fe, provides a luminous welcome with its wall fountain.

facing, top: Wood, water, sky, and fresh air rejuvenate naturally at Ten Thousand Waves Japanese Spa and Retreat, Santa Fe, New Mexico.

facing, bottom: Dappled reflections soothe, in an outdoor hot tub at Ten Thousand Waves Japanese Spa and Retreat, Santa Fe, New Mexico.

INSTANT ENERGY TRICKS FOR PERKING UP

• Sip six to eight ounces of purified, room temperature water to spark up energy transmissions between neural cells. You'll really feel the difference, especially if your foot, leg, and arm muscles have been cramped up in tensed positions.

• Purposefully walk up and down stairs instead of taking the escalator or elevator. Focus on the present moment. Imagine your body cells gaining more power with every step you take, with the new infusion of oxygen intake empowering every cell of your body. Climbing stairs also provides strength training for endurance, quite different from aerobic activities such as jogging or running.

• Go outside your home or office cubicle and walk briskly around the block a couple of times to pump new oxygen into your body cells to reinvigorate tired, old energy. Do not be distracted by thoughts as you gradually pick up speed by focusing on your pace and breathing. Your inner pilot will intuitively guide you to pick up a comfy tempo, depending on your gait and breathing. Move your arms forwards and backwards at right angles and imagine tired energy and stress falling off with each movement. Consciously reenter your workspace with a lighter step and a more positive attitude.

• Take an ethereal twinkie break. Rather than reaching for a calorie-laden Twinkie-like snack, pull out instead a pocket twinkie meditation. Sit up straight. Close your eyes. Focus on your breathing—breathe in deeply and slowly, hold your breath for two counts, then exhale gently. Repeat a few times. You begin to loosen up, becoming more aware of your energy levels recharging. When you relax and stay calm, your muscles are able to load up on positive energy again. (The obverse is true. Negative energy charged with resentment, anger, and depression debilitates muscles—in effect paralyzing the person with hopelessness.)

a stagnant pool), water is evident not only in bodily functions making up 65 to 70 percent of the human body, but also in psychologically de-stressing bathers at home or nurturing camaraderie and friendship at a *sento*, or public bath, in Japan.

In Europe, healing waters of Mediterranean mineral baths enjoyed by the Romans and the Greeks also hark back thousands of years, giving rise to the Latin *sanus per aquum* (health through water), now shortened to the common term, *spa*.

The Italians call it *terme*, or "taking to the waters," for healing and rejuvenating purposes. Similarly, the Japanese take to the waters at the *onsen*, at over 2,500 natural mineral springs (either hot or cold) locations dotting the islands of Japan.

Yoshi Nakano, a shiatsu instructor from Tucson, Arizona, explains that urban Japanese families travel as family units to rural villages for meaningful reunions at the end of the year. It symbolically marks, "a washing away of old energy, to welcome in the New Year with the whole extended family sharing in a joyful celebration of the new," Nakano notes, "and is especially significant in a Shinto culture that honors purification of body, mind, and spirit."

For Nakano, the pilgrimage-like expedition to visit an *onsen* fosters a sense of "coming home, in being taken by the mineral waters to safety, and away from fear. You just let drop all your defenses." How so? "Because you are embraced by nature in the company of others in a deeper way. It's an awareness of seeing others as spiritual beings, and not just as human beings. It's a shared sense of cleansing your spirit, not just washing your body clean," says Nakano, in describing how ritual purification via the public bath is, after all, a very pure experience in Japan, even though bathers are in the buff, save for a small towel.[1]

Apart from the spiritual, Nakano says the eastern health-care approach is one that is rooted in preventive measures. And, a highly practical measure—one that is "not fooled by symptoms after they have manifested," he says. Like the Europeans, the Japanese take to the waters to purify body-mind-spirit regularly before pathogenesis sets in.

In the American Southwest, when warring tribes met at hot springs, it was a call to lay down arms. It was an opportunity to reconcile and recuperate before moving on. The world-renowned Ojo Caliente Spa north of Santa Fe, New Mexico, is the only place in the world bubbling up four different mineral waters, all

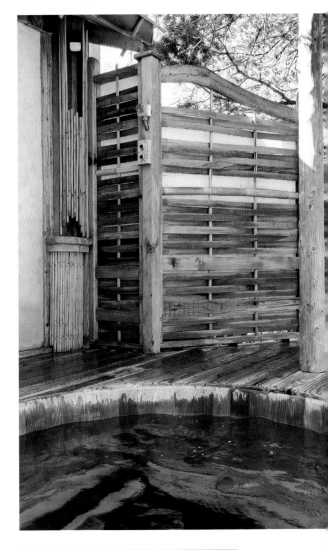

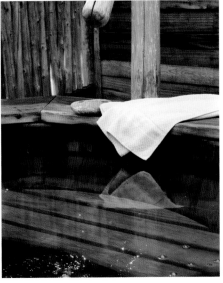

[1] Japanese spa etiquette requires the towel to be either folded over and placed on the head or by the side of the pool—not dipping into the spa water shared by others.

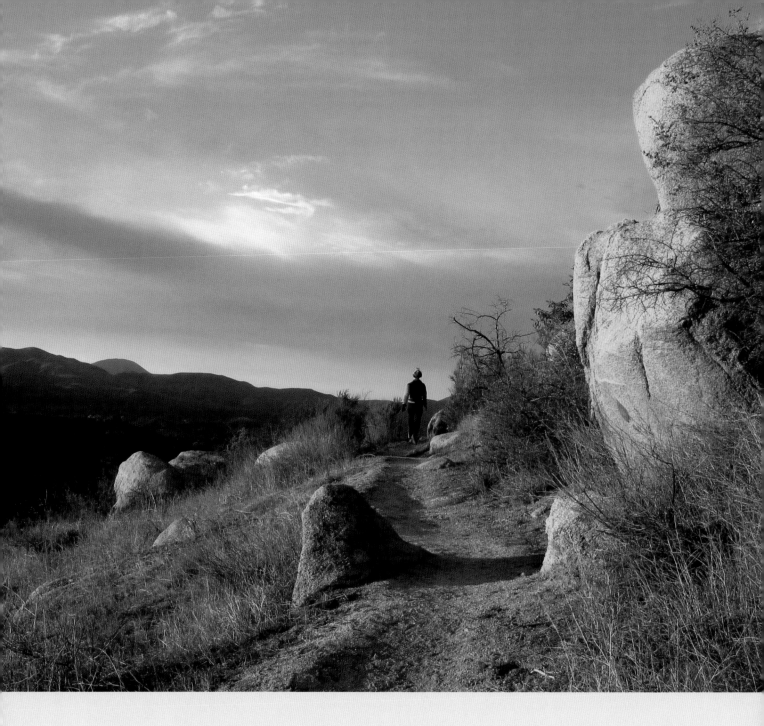

PRACTICAL TIPS FOR GENERATING POSITIVE ENERGY

By Jenean LaRoche, Spa Director, Nob Hill Spa, The Huntington Hotel, San Francisco

- Get eight hours of beauty sleep.
- Exercise regularly.
- Engage in a stress-reduction activity, such as meditation.
- Invest time and energy with your skin care, and use products relevant to your skin type.
- Don't smoke.
- Maintain a healthy diet—don't drink soda; eat five to six servings of fruits and veggies daily.
- Find a place to volunteer that is a good fit for your interests.
- Take adult education classes for fun.
- Get a dog.

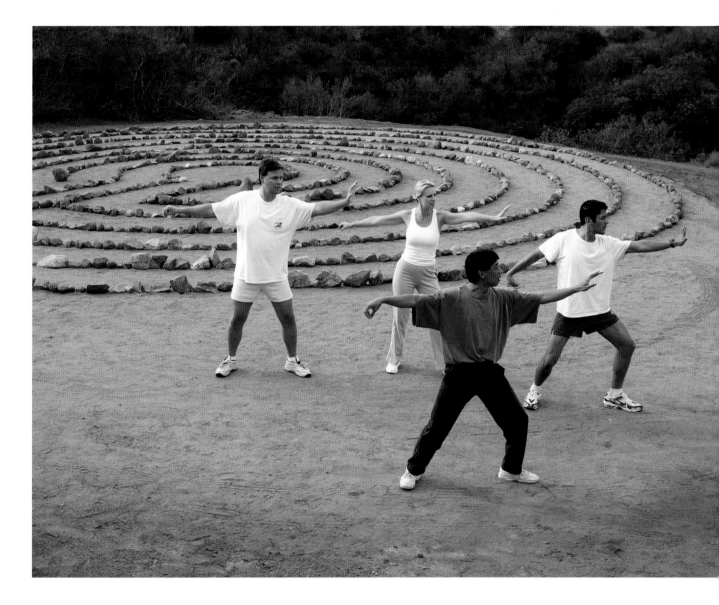

at one spot. The Ancients built their Pueblos overlooking these sacred hot springs, forebears of today's Tewa Indians, and named the healing waters *Posi* or *Poseuinge*, "village at the place of the green bubbling hot springs."

Christened by sixteenth-century conquistador Cabezade de Vaca as Ojo Calient, (meaning *hot springs*), the waters thrilled and rejuvenated the Spaniards with four different mineral springs—iron, arsenic, lithia, and soda. Over four hundred years later, many continue coming to take these waters, with Ojo Caliente gushing up over 100,000 steaming gallons daily from a subterranean volcanic aquifer, healing those who drink, bath in, and take, these waters.

facing: **Out on the trails for an early hike at Rancho la Puerta.** (Courtesy photo)

Tai chi and walking the labyrinth reenergize at Cal-a-Vie. (Courtesy photo)

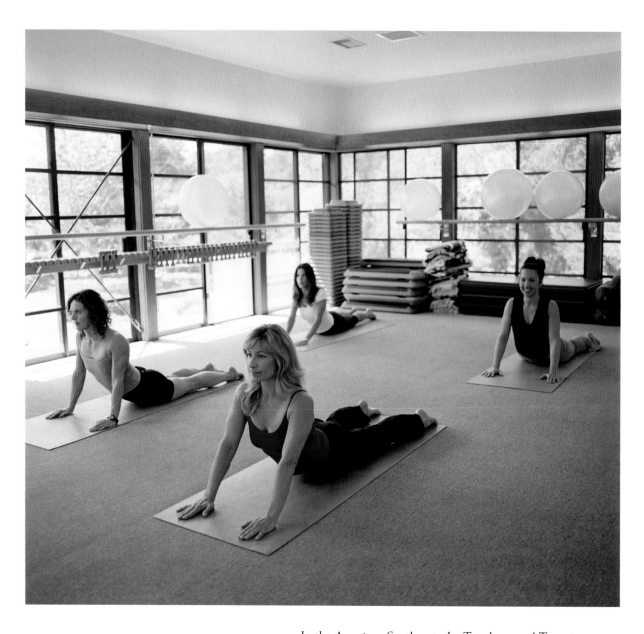

In the American Southeast, the Tocobaga and Timucuan Indians enjoyed the hot springs at Safety Harbor, Florida, for over two thousand years. In May 1539, Spanish adventurer Hernando De Soto arrived. Although unsuccessful in finding either gold or silver, De Soto declared a most valuable discovery in these curative hot springs, which he christened Espiritu Santo, and dubbed them, "The Fountain of Youth."[2]

Still wondering why nature's minerals, oxygen, and water figure so prominently in promoting a sense of well-being, while maintaining optimal health? Try taking the waters regularly at a mineral spring and tap into Nature's naturally healing elixirs.

A yoga glass at Golden Door spa.
(Courtesy photo)

[2] Since the 1850s, Safety Harbor Resort and Spa has been renowned worldwide for its healing waters.

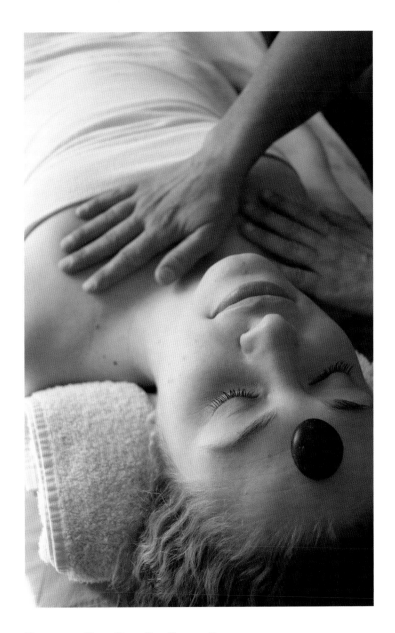

About 25 percent of U.S. workers in the private sector do not get any paid vacation time, the Bureau of Labor Statistics reports. An additional 33 percent will take only a seven-day vacation, including a weekend.

The Travel Industry Association, the largest trade group representing the industry, found that the average American expects his or her longest summer trip to last six nights. And it takes three days just to begin to unwind, experts say.

—Reported by Timothy Egan in "The Rise of Shrinking-Vacation Syndrome," *New York Times*, August 20, 2006

Designing Your Own Spa Fitness Programs

Destination spas design workout-reward systems that enhance cardiovascular and strength training by sweating out toxins and toning muscles. Early-morning strenuous hikes up and down hills take a gradual getting used to over the course of a week's stay. But the payoff is huge—the body struggles to adjust initially, then learns to capitalize on the payload with oxygenated cells delivering even more energy and endurance.

This is followed by salubrious treats in the afternoon, to rebalance the body with massages, herbal body wraps that purport to draw out more toxins, and soothing facials.

At Ojo Caliente, hot stones and touch therapies maximize energy flows. (Courtesy photo)

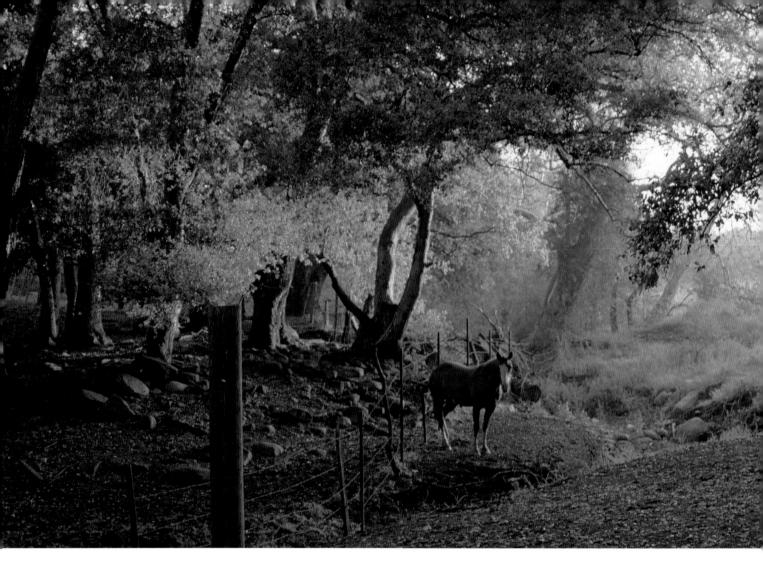

You, too, can develop your own spa programs at home and at work to arrive at similar energizing levels of rewards and deep satisfaction that comes from exercising well. Bicycling, jogging, and vigorous walking to work or to catch the train or bus can count as morning workouts. If you can shower at work, all the better.

And, in the course of ten work days, schedule a series of different, one-hour rewards in the afternoon—pedicure, manicure, hair appointment, facial, bodywork or massage, dance/yoga/nia/ pilates class, window shopping, high tea with a friend, art gallery opening, food sampling at the farmers' market, or wine tasting at a Whole Foods Market—while varying the times each day, for variety's sake.

All of this amounts to lots of moving around, and enjoying emotional experiences that enliven with gusto, good will, and gustatory delight. In a nutshell, this is how spas pamper guests with fun vignettes of work-play experiences broken up into bite-sized portions that anyone can innovate, expand on, and personalize, according to their own interests.

Early-morning hikes below the oak trees at Rancho la Puerta. (Courtesy photo)

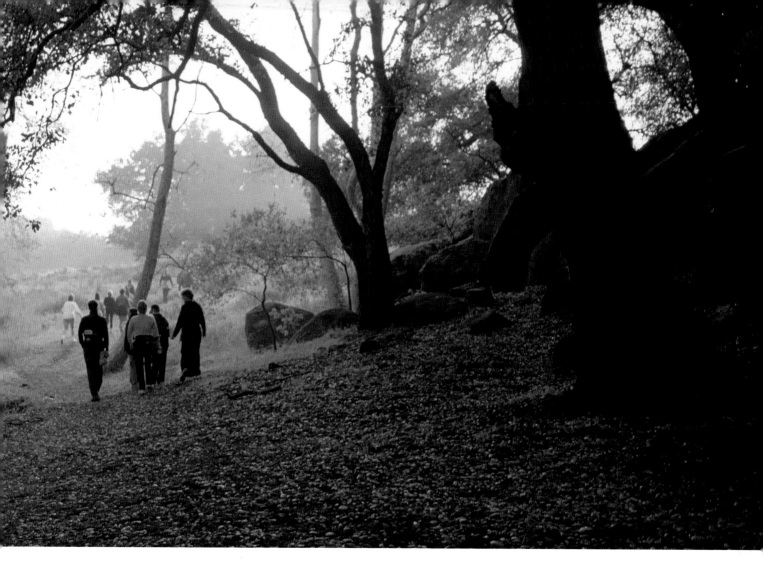

LIFESTYLE CHANGES REVERBERATE FROM SPA TO HOME

By Sandy Novak, Seattle, Washington

One of my goals when I returned to Rancho La Puerta (a destination spa in Tecate, Mexico) was to gain more stamina for hiking. In anticipation of this, I walked more, and took on routes with challenging hills. When I got to Rancho, I was able to complete Alex's Oak Tree Hike (two and three-quarter miles) and several other hikes—which I could not do a year ago.

Each year, my husband and I go on a camping trip with friends. Usually, I struggle to keep up with the group on our hikes. This year, I was able to manage the hiking quite easily. Did that ever feel good!

My next adventure is to go with thirteen other women to hike the Camino de Santiago in northern Spain.

Last year, I retired from my job. I have now joined a gym. I want to focus on upper body strength and weight training. I know I would not be conscious of these healthy exercise needs if it wasn't for Rancho.

A SEDENTARY LIFESTYLE AND THE pH FACTOR

By Yvonne Nienstadt, Nutrition Director, Rancho La Puerta Fitness Resort and Spa, Tecate, Mexico

A normal pH of all tissues and fluids in the human body, except for stomach and skin, is slightly alkaline. The term *pH* stands for "potential" of "Hydrogen," to indicate the amount of hydrogen ions in a particular solution. More hydrogen ions in a solution make it more acidic, while fewer hydrogen ions make it more alkaline. pH is measured on a scale of 0 to 14, with 7 being neutral.

The most critical pH balance for the human body is in the blood. All other organs and fluids will fluctuate in their range to keep the blood strictly between 7.35 and 7.45. Through homeostasis (or the rhythm of staying balanced), the body makes constant adjustments in tissue and fluid pH to maintain this narrow pH range in the blood.

Lifestyle factors contribute to acidity in the blood. This happens when a sedentary lifestyle sets in, or the person gets dehydrated, becomes mentally and/or physically stressed out, and lives in an environmentally polluted area.

The blood turns acidic too, when too much is consumed of refined sugars, alcohol, soft drinks, processed foods, meats, and fried foods.

There are serious consequences when the body gets too acidic. For example, blood will balance out its pH level at all costs, by borrowing alkalinizing minerals such as calcium and magnesium from bones and tissues.

That's when symptoms start showing up, such as indigestion, heart burn, acid reflux, poor metabolism, weight gain or difficulty losing weight, mineral deficiencies, constipation, fatigue, brain fog, frequent urination, hypoglycemia, hormonal imbalances, and toxins building up in tissues contributing to sore muscles and joints, which sets the stage for infections to proliferate, and degenerative diseases to set in.

According to Dr. Theodore A. Baroody, author of *Alkalize or Die* (Holographic Health Press, 1991), we age because we accumulate toxic acidic wastes. Eating more fruits, vegetables, and whole grains mitigates acid toxicity; while refined foods, animal protein, alcohol, coffee, and smoking, exacerbate it.

It is therefore important to be aware of acidity levels in the body and the pH factor. Short of getting Dr. Baroody's book, an abbreviated list of alkaline-acid foods is available at: http://www.focus-on-nutrition.com/FoodpH.shtml.

An exercise room at Rancho la Puerta. (Courtesy photo)

facing: Cal-a-Vie's Jacuzzi room in the Bath House calms with a muted palette, redolent in casual elegance typical of French country style (although the blue-white trompe l'oeil mural is Portuguese). (Courtesy photo)

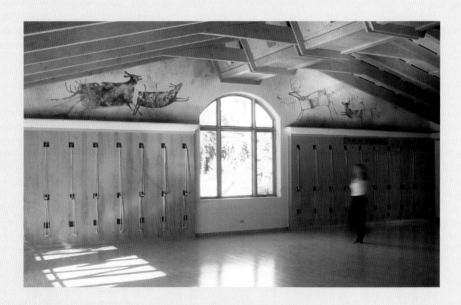

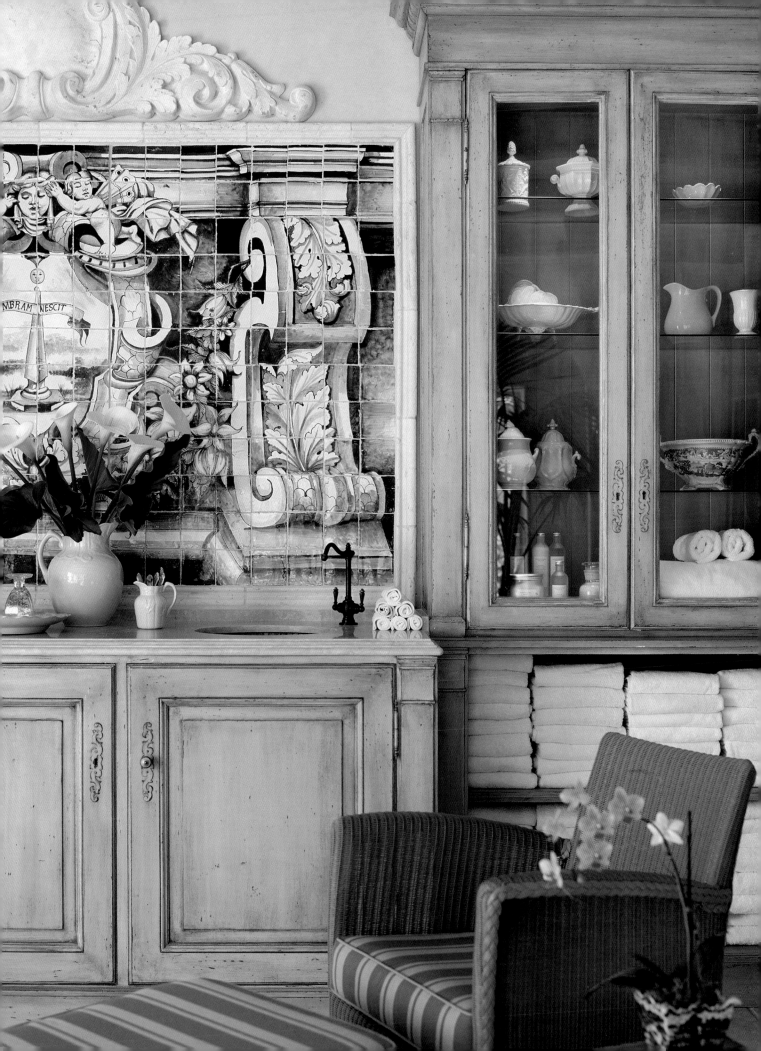

In a week or two, depending on the individual, the gains are remarkably noticeable—you've earned more energy to expend and are therefore more productive, your body feels lighter without being sluggish, and most of all, an upbeat demeanor emerges to face challenges in surmounting them easily.

While at it, enjoy the myriad benefits of staying fit and healthy by:

- experimenting and innovating with different forms of physical exercise you find fun—walking, jogging, nias, dancing, bicycling, or swimming—a smorgasbord of cross training to give various muscles a good workout;

- consciously incorporating the two major elemental forces of nature—oxygen and water—into your routines; and

- getting plenty of rest in between, as well as eating a nutritious diet that promotes alkaline levels for your body's circulatory systems to function optimally.

The silent blessings of Mount Kuchumaa in the morning light inspires guests to walk and hike during the early hours at Rancho la Puerta. (Courtesy photo)

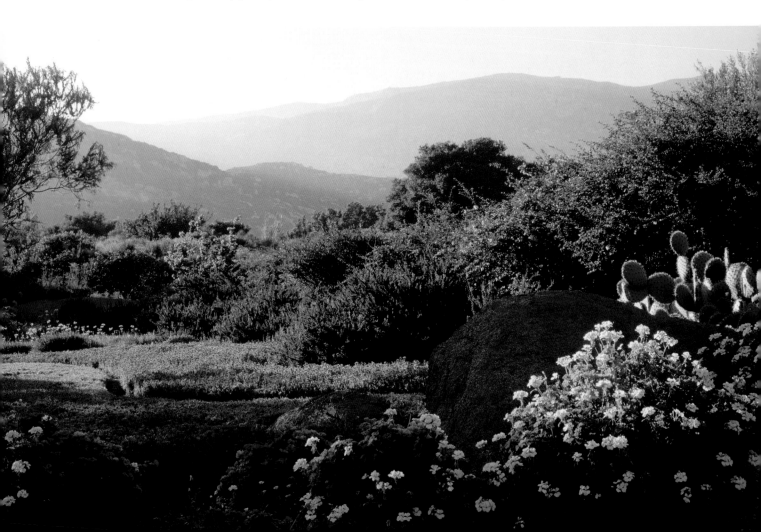

THE POWER OF SOULFUL GRACE:
TWICE-BLESSED FOOD IS MORE NOURISHING

Many families today still find time to offer heartfelt thanks before enjoying a meal together. This silent moment of gratitude, or the act of saying grace, serves to nourish twofold by subtly transforming energy with our sincere intentions.

First, it invites quiet time to calm down the mind and body—to focus on taking time to enjoy eating and sharing, thus assisting the digestive juices to assimilate food properly.

Second, the diner has the power to elevate eating and dining with a positive attitude to invoke Light to bless the food—a divinely nourishing experience that adds to a higher level of feeling satisfied with food intake.

In India, the invocation, *Annam Brahma* means: God is Food; Food is God. The gifts of nature are exactly so—from the source divine, and therefore a meaningful gesture and tribute to the source in acknowledging its powerful, yet subtle, force in nurturing us with good health and plenitude.

Similarly, it helps to prepare food with a loving and dynamic consciousness to pass along these positive vibrations to diners. Or, cook with a caring and tender demeanor when preparing food for the elderly, as my meditation master, Sri Chinmoy, suggests.

When you become your heart's gratitude,
God becomes your life's plenitude.

—Sri Chinmoy

TWO JAPANESE SECRETS FOR POSITIVE ENERGY
TRANSFORMATION

By Yoshi Nakano, Shiatsu Instructor, Tucson, Arizona

1. **A Peaceful Conversion.** When you relax and calm down your mind and emotions, your lymphatic and cardiovascular circulatory systems become more alkaline, which enables your blood to release melatonin, which in turn relaxes your muscles. When lymphatic drainage is working properly, toxins are washed away and eliminated easily. When the cardiovascular system is operating maximally, oxygen intake increases, converting to more energy for your body's needs. When your circulatory systems are working optimally, your immune system is enhanced—and your body is powerfully poised to battle pathogens and disease-causing organisms, which are all around us.

2. **A Culinary Conversion.** In Japanese culture, food is medicine. In Japan, we ask the chef on a daily basis, "What is *shun* food for today?" *Shun* means seasonal. Traditionally, the Japanese have noticed how environmental energy fluctuates and changes about every ten days. Since our bodies have to acclimate to the seasons, more than half the battle to stay healthy is won when we eat seasonally, in tune with Nature's offerings. Eating *shun* is eating the very best for the current season.

In Japanese culture, food is medicine.

—Yoshi Nakano

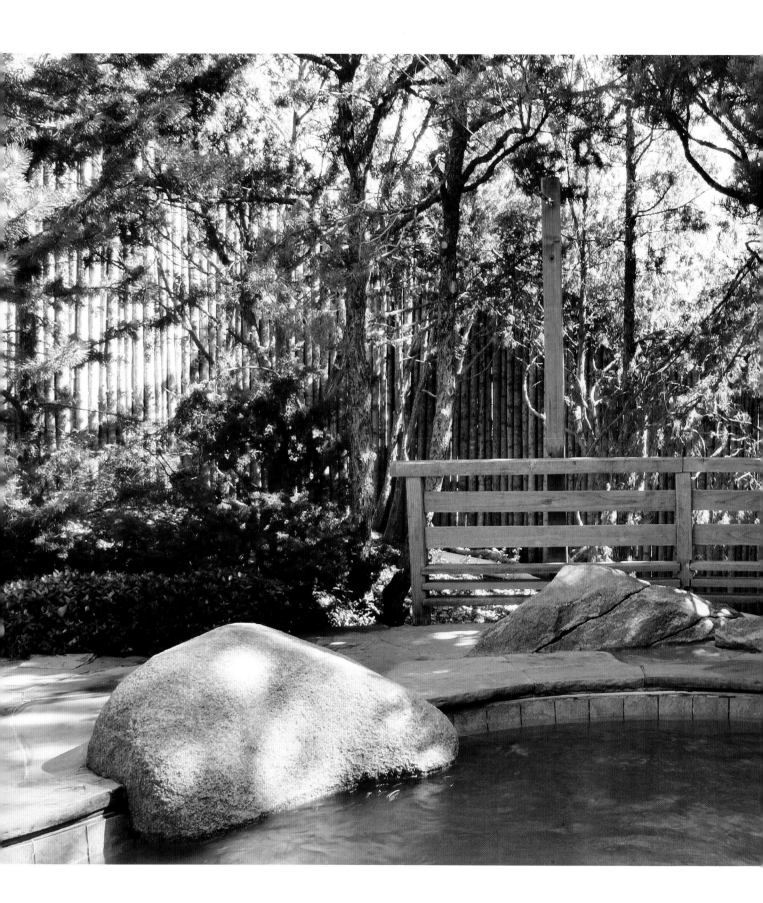

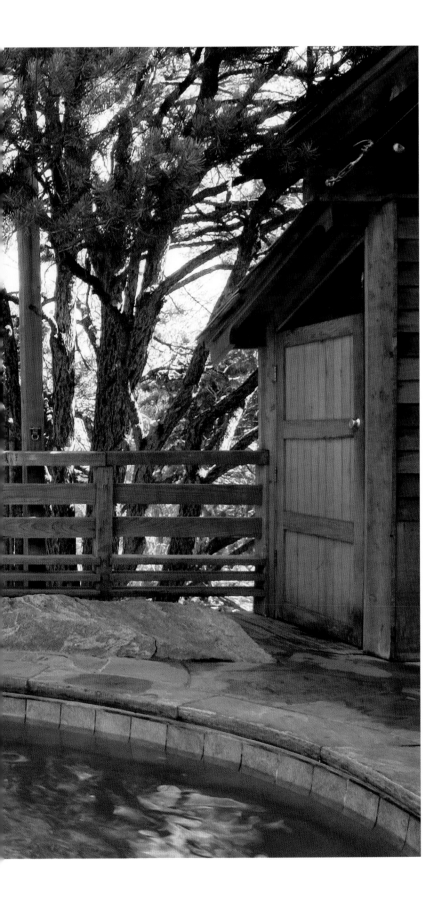

The secluded Waterfall outdoor tub basks in nature's cocoon of trees, coyote fence, rocks, and sky at Ten Thousand Waves Japanese Spa and Retreat, Santa Fe, New Mexico.

CHAPTER SIX

ENJOYING
SPA CUISINE

As my awareness grew about the role of food as medicine, I observed that many health problems seemed intertwined with the stresses of daily life. These include worries about one's job or money, tension and even the stress created by eating the wrong kinds of food and improper food combining.

The golden keys to health lie in getting in touch with your inner self and in seeing the process of healing as a useful means of learning about your own unique needs.

—Dr. Vasant Lad, Founder of The Ayurvedic Institute, Albuquerque, New Mexico, in *Ayurvedic Cooking for Self-Healing*

One of the more joyful gifts of living well is eating well. This hearty activity of the table not only nurtures family ties and friendship among strangers, it also nourishes deeply those who take time to taste every delicious morsel in a well-planned and balanced meal—by bestowing good health through the grace of heavenly eating. Every meal prepared with a loving consciousness and served graciously, blesses diners with the indelible stamp of divine delight.

The unfortunate upshot of overindulgence in gustatory adventures can, of course, tilt the scales to anomalous ways affecting the physical body and the emotional mind.

Foraging at Fat Farms

In the early 1980s, a proliferation of fat farms tried to abjure those tortured with gustatory remorse, some semblance of solace. Those who docked in at fat farms were the overweight who had, of course, the means to be catered to in spa-like settings to whittle down excess pounds. Sadly, fat farms as a genre came to earn unwelcome reputations of spa cuisine with bland, tasteless victuals, and mean-sized portions that failed to satisfy.

Taking time to pause for an energy drink at Cornelia Day Resort & Spa.
(Courtesy photo)

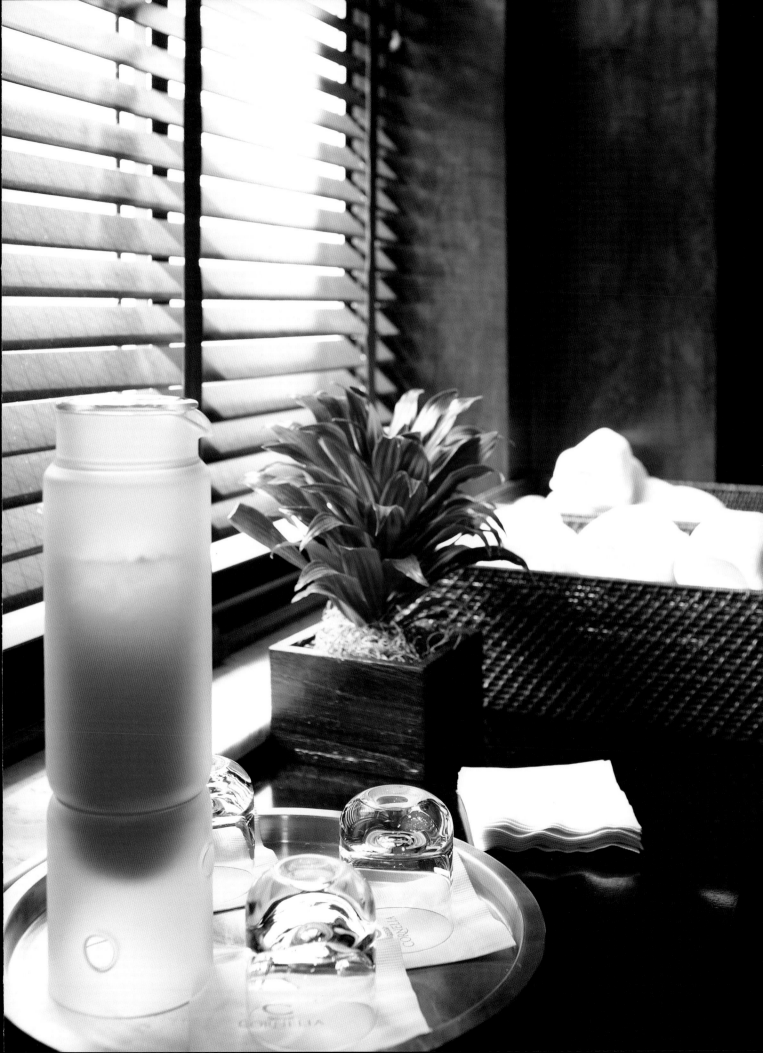

Cal-a-Vie's Frozen Raspberry Mousse

From Executive Chef Steve Pernetti

3 cups frozen raspberries

3 tablespoons honey

3/4 ripe banana

1 teaspoon pure vanilla extract

1/2 cup vanilla protein powder

1/4 cup sweetener

1/4 cup fresh orange juice

Combine all ingredients in a chilled food processor; process for about 5 minutes or until mixture becomes thick and smooth. Divide into 8 chilled dessert cups; garnish with mint and fresh raspberries.

Serve as soon as possible or refreeze and scoop it out like ice cream. Serves 8.

So, it was little wonder that fat farms did not garner the support they had so heroically set out to do, to earn investors and owners humongous returns on their investments. Fat farm attendees—frantic though they were to live off the fatuous notion that such diet spas could shed off excess fat in a week two—eventually gave up on the paltry servings and unsatisfactory lack of comfort food dished up without their preferred buttered drippings.

But thank goodness, common sense finally dawned; as is often the case when dissatisfaction rears its head, and the mouth is ready to forgo chewing on more drivel.

Today's Healthy and Heavenly Spa Cuisine

Enter desirable destination spa meals of the late 1980s and 1990s—served with élan on fine china and larger-sized portions made with organic ingredients, sans heavy meats. The new millennium of lighter meals prepared from vegetables and fruits redolent with their still-fresh flavors earned honors on the spa menu, at both destination and day spas.

Cal-a-Vie[1], French for "California life," is a salubrious destination spa that dishes up hearty portions of delicious gourmet lunches on a lovely patio by a gently splashing mini waterfall. More sedate breakfasts and dinners are served in the Provencal-style dining room with glorious views of the property, which includes a French stone chapel built in 1615. This jewel was shipped over from Burgundy, France, by Cal-a-Vie owners Terri and John Havens, and reassembled brick by brick, now serenely crowning its own hilltop. Evening meditations in this chapel divinely transport spa guests to other realms of consciousness.

Meals at this destination spa offer generous servings of fresh greens for entrées and fruit for dessert, lightly tossed with flavorful herbs such as mint and dashes of spices (cumin and coriander)—culinary magic that robust eaters cannot turn down, especially after their well-earned morning workouts.

As Dr. Dean Ornish makes the same case in his compelling book, *Eat More, Weigh Less* (HarperTorch, 2001), it is no coincidence that the most hearty meal of the day at Cal-a-Vie is lunch, the better to work off calories in the course of the day's activities.

Steve Pernetti, Cal-a-Vie's head chef since 1994, customizes individual menus for guests according to their caloric intakes. Typically, 1,200 to 1,400 calories per day is the norm for female guests. Pernetti shares some of his secrets for healthy spa cuisine:

[1] Located forty miles north of San Diego, California, Cal-a-Vie is embraced by undulating hills and panoramic vistas, www.calavie.com.

- Base protein portion size on the size of your palm, not your hand.
- Use a ratio of 60-20-20 for complex carbohydrates-protein-fats in your menu if you're planning on increased physical activities (as during your stay at this spa) for the extra carbs to fuel your workouts.
- Honor your cravings to prevent binging out. Instead of three main meals a day, enjoy healthy snacks throughout—such as grilled veggies lightly dressed with sea salt or Braggs' amino seasoning, nuts, and fresh fruit.
- Keep out butters and heavy oils so the fresh produce play out their flavors better.
- Eat with the seasons and go organic whenever you can.
- Don't get stuck on the same foods every day—try new variations and have fun mixing different flavors.
- Be sure to drink lots of water, which takes the edge off hunger.

Before coming to Cal-a-Vie, Pernetti was sous chef at another stellar destination spa, Golden Door,[2] which opened in 1958 in Escondido, California. Michel Stroot was Golden Door's executive chef for over three decades, ever since he assumed the mantle in 1973, at founder Deborah Szekely's invitation.

Stroot defines spa cuisine for guests in his cookbook, *The Golden Door Cooks Light & Easy* (Gibbs Smith, 2003). "It wasn't a cuisine of denial or abstinence. For many guests, it was all about rediscovering the great flavors and freshness of childhood days spent on farms, in small towns, and even in great cities before the days of chain markets and restaurants. The big difference was the lack of butters and other animal fats common to classical cooking. It was, in a word, *light*," Stroot explains.

Inspired, Stroot and Szekely created menus that capture the beauty and flavor of classical cuisine, but innovative and light, in touch with the seasons, and—delicious. Since Stroot's retirement, Dean Rucker continues to draw returning guests for the delectable dining treats that Golden Door is known for.

Golden Door's nutritionist, Dr. Wendy Bazilian, makes the case for drinking adequate amounts of filtered or spring water daily, because every bodily function depends on water as a key nutrient, from mobility in the joints and ease of bodily movements and digestion, to the eyelids blinking. In developing menus, Bazilian works from plant-based dishes in accommodating individual guest preferences to celebrate good food with abundance—an abundance she equates with "the diversity of enjoying how good food is plated and presented, how it tastes with complementary flavors and textures, and not just portion size."

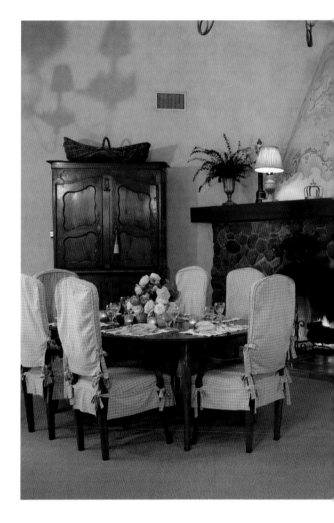

Cal-a-Vie's Provençal-style dining room serves low-calorie haute cuisine prepared by executive chef Steve Pernetti and his culinary team. (Courtesy photo)

---

[2] Golden Door was razed for highway expansion in the early '70s. Reincarnated in 1975 as a *honjin*, or ancient Japanese country-style inn, Golden Door accepts only forty guests for a seven-day stay. See www.goldendoor.com.

Eggplant "Caviar" with Purple Potatoes

Black sesame seeds give this eggplant "caviar" a look that approximates the real thing. Pairing the slate-colored eggplant with purple potatoes produces an appetizer that looks as good as it tastes. The eggplant can also be served as a dip for crudités or with tortilla chips.

1 large eggplant
Canola oil in a spray bottle, or 1 teaspoon canola oil
5 medium purple potatoes (about 2 pounds)
1/2 cup finely chopped fresh parsley
1 tablespoon finely chopped capers drained
1 tablespoon olive oil
2 teaspoons balsamic vinegar
2 teaspoons fresh lemon juice
1 teaspoon minced garlic
1/2 teaspoon ground cumin
1/2 teaspoon freshly ground black pepper
1/2 teaspoon salt, or to taste
1 1/2 tablespoons sesame seeds, preferably black
Vegetable oil in a spray bottle, or 1 teaspoon vegetable oil
Fresh chervil sprigs for garnish

Preheat the oven to 350 degrees F. Spray or brush the eggplant with canola oil, pierce with a fork, and place into a shallow baking dish. Roast for about 1 hour, or until soft, turning once.

Meanwhile, place the potatoes into a medium-sized pot with enough water to cover, and bring to a boil. Boil for about 15 minutes, or until fork-tender but still firm. Remove from the heat, drain and let cool. Slice the cooled potatoes, with skins on, into 1/4-inch rounds; set aside.

When the eggplant is done, cut it in half lengthwise and let it cool. Scrape the eggplant pulp away from the peel, and place the pulp into a blender or food processor fitted with a metal blade. Add the parsley, capers, olive oil, balsamic vinegar, lemon juice, garlic, cumin, black pepper, and salt; pulse to a coarse consistency, then transfer to a mixing bowl.

Set a small, dry nonstick pan over medium heat. Add the sesame seeds and toast lightly, stirring often, for 2 to 3 minutes. Stir the toasted seeds into the eggplant mixture.

Spray or grease a separate nonstick pan with vegetable oil and set over medium-high heat. Place the potatoes into the pan in a single layer and sear for 2 minutes on each side, or until light brown. Remove and let cool.

To serve, place about 5 or 6 potato slices onto an appetizer plate. Top each with 2 teaspoons of the eggplant "caviar" and garnish with sprigs of chervil. Assemble 5 more plates. Makes 6 servings.

facing: Eggplant "Caviar" with Purple Potatoes, Golden Door spa. (Courtesy photo)

Golden Door Potassium Broth

4 cups vegetable trimmings such as celery, onion, carrot, cabbage,
    parsley stems, basil, and 2 crushed garlic cloves
2 pounds plum tomatoes (12 to 14 tomatoes, quartered) or one
    29-ounce can crushed plum tomatoes
10 cups water

In a small soup pot, combine vegetable trimmings, plum tomatoes, and water. Bring to a boil, reduce heat, and simmer about 45 minutes. Strain, and discard the solids.

Season to taste. Serve broth hot or cold. Good source of vitamin C, vitamin A, and potassium. Makes 12 servings.

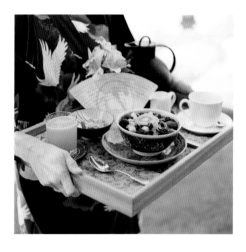

above: Serving up a tasty, healthy breakfast at Golden Door spa. (Courtesy photo)

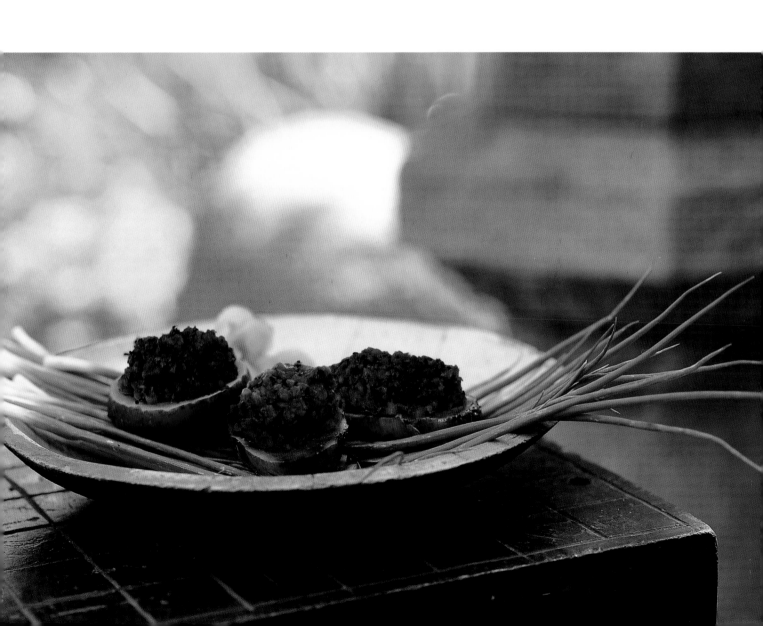

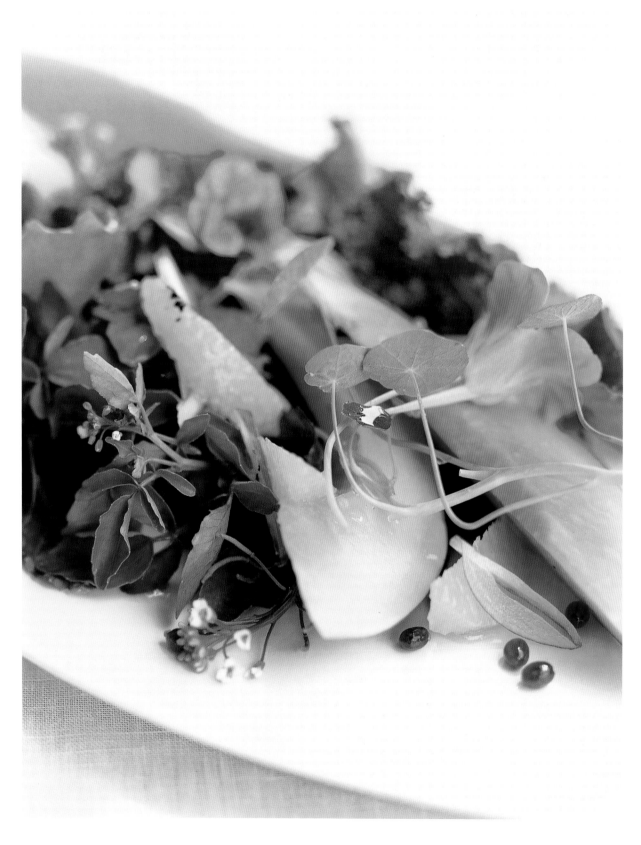

Papaya, Orange, and Bermuda Onion Salad,
Golden Door spa. (Courtesy photo)

Ginger, Peanut, and Cilantro Sauce and Dressing

This dressing is one of the most popular at the Golden Door. It's one of those multitasking condiments that can be used as a dipping sauce for baked wontons or vegetables; as a sauce for grilled poultry, seafood, or meat dishes; or as a dressing for all kinds of salads. Keep in mind that as ginger gets older, it tends to get stringy; if you can find it, you can substitute galangal, ginger's Southeast Asian cousin. Its texture is less stringy.

1 1/2 tablespoons minced fresh gingerroot

1 tablespoon rice vinegar

1/4 cup fresh orange juice

1 tablespoon fresh lime juice

1 teaspoon Vietnamese chili sauce

2 tablespoons chunky peanut butter

1 tablespoon honey

2 tablespoons water

4 sprigs fresh cilantro

Combine the ginger, vinegar, orange juice, lime juice, chili sauce, peanut butter, honey and water in a blender or food processor fitted with a metal blade; process until smooth. Add the cilantro sprigs and pulse to combine. This dressing can be kept in the refrigerator, covered, for 5 days. Makes 1 cup.

Papaya, Orange, and Bermuda Onion Salad

1/2 small Bermuda onion, thinly sliced

1 tablespoon sherry vinegar

1/4 cup fresh orange juice

1 tablespoon fresh lime juice

1 tablespoon olive oil

2 oranges, peeled, pith removed and separated into segments

4 cups mixed greens, washed and patted dry

1 large papaya, peeled, seeded, and sliced lengthwise into 12 strips

4 nasturtium flowers, optional

In a small mixing bowl, combine the Bermuda onion and sherry vinegar; marinate for 15 minutes.

Prepare the dressing by whisking together the orange juice, lime juice, and olive oil in a small bowl. Using a sharp knife, cut the outer membrane from the orange segments. Place equal portions of the mixed greens onto chilled salad plates. Arrange the sliced papaya around the greens and top with the orange segments and marinated onions. Drizzle the dressing over the top and garnish with the nasturtiums, if using. Makes 4 servings.

Mango-Tahini Dressing

Tart-sweet mangoes get a nutty infusion from tahini, the paste made from ground sesame seeds. The tahini is so rich you only need a tablespoon, which keeps the fat content of this dressing to a minimum. Use it to dress chicken salad, jicama salad, or grilled fish or lamb.

1 ripe mango, peeled, pitted, and diced
1 tablespoon minced shallot
1 tablespoon tahini
3 tablespoons fresh lime juice
1 teaspoon Champagne vinegar or white balsamic vinegar
1/2 cup water
1 teaspoon minced lime zest

Combine the mango, shallot, tahini, lime juice, vinegar, and water in a blender or food processor fitted with a metal blade; process until smooth. Transfer to a bowl and stir in the minced lime zest. This dressing can be kept in the refrigerator, covered, for 4 to 5 days. Makes 2 cups.

All Recipes from *The Golden Door Cooks Light & Easy* by Chef Michel Stroot (Gibbs Smith, Publisher, 2003).

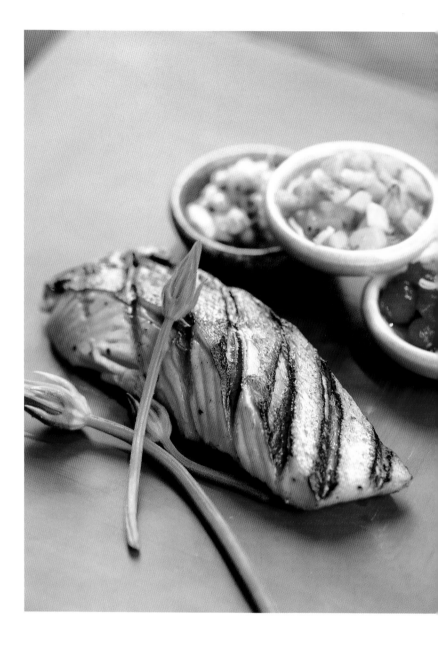

Golden Gazpacho, Golden Door spa.
(Courtesy photo)

When Deborah Szekely[3] started Golden Door spa, she brought with her a wealth of experiences from having started with her late husband, Edmond, the first modern destination spa. Rancho La Puerta,[4] renowned the world over as "the mother of modern destination spas," is three miles south of the U.S.-Mexican border in Tecate.

Back when Rancho opened in 1940, guests actually helped milk goats for their victuals. But more than six decades later,

[3] Many people do not know that Deborah Szekely wrote *the* Congressional management guide, *Setting Course*, prompted by her only bid for public office that ended in failure. Finding no publication existed to help freshmen members of Congress transition to their new responsibilities, she wrote this book in 1983; now into its ninth edition. Szekely's amazing comeback genius continues to fuel her other civic activities.

[4] A neat activity is eating with heightened awareness at the Meditation Dinner, www.ranch(olapuerta.com

Creative Chef (yes, that's his correct title) Jesus Gonzalez proudly dishes up "about 90 percent organic fare for breakfast, lunch, and dinner," harvested from their two-and-a-half-acre organic garden, the result of Szekely's daughter's green thumb. Sarah Livia Brightwood oversees Rancho's organic garden from England, where she now lives with her family. Both women have broken ground for a cooking school at the garden.

Gonzalez's gustatory credo is "prepared from the garden to the plate." (While at Rancho, I was momentarily floored by how flavorful strawberries in May can be.) Nurtured in an environment where creativity flourishes, Gonzalez had started at Golden Door as a dishwasher; fifteen years later, he was invited to head Rancho's culinary team.[5]

Another cooking insight from Gonzalez: "While fresh, organic produce is important for healthy eating, I also find that food is a 100 percent influenced by the cook's emotions. That's why we like to work harmoniously as a team in our kitchen," he says.

Rancho's sumptuous breakfast and lunch buffets are legendary. Many guests are oblivious to the absence of meat— that is, until dinnertime, when seafood (the only meat served) appears as an entrée selection for the sit-down repast in the *sala grande*.

Also a noteworthy observation: do the predominantly plant-based Rancho menus keep the *cucaracha* (cockroaches) away? They were certainly absent guests, compared to other tropical establishments where one would invariably have to share space and crumbs with.

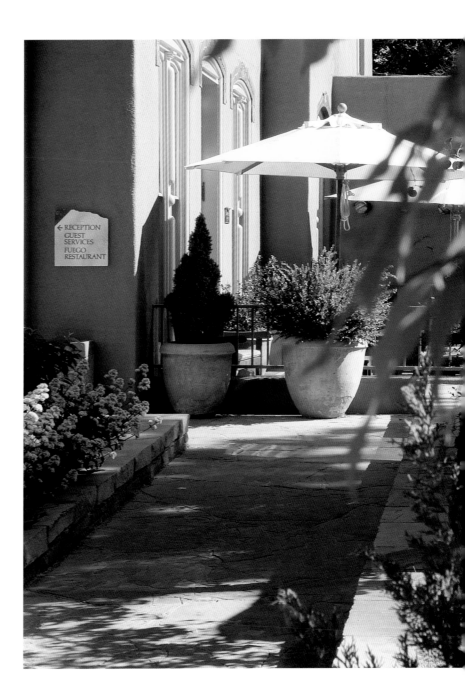

A refreshing breezeway connects Avanyu Spa at La Posada de Santa Fe to its historic Staab House.

[5] Golden Door was sold to Wyndham Hotels in 1998, which later resold it to the Luxury Report chain. Since then, Golden Door is trademarked to other properties in the chain offering their own spa services.

Recipes from Rancho la Puerta

All recipes by Creative Chef Jesus Gonzalez of the Culinary Team at Rancho La Puerta Fitness Resort & Spa, Tecate, Mexico

Spanakopita

1/2 teaspoon olive oil

1 medium onion, chopped

1/2 teaspoon minced garlic

6 cups fresh spinach

2 to 2 1/2 cups fresh kale or chard (or more spinach)

1/4 cup fresh chopped parsley

1 1/2 to 2 tablespoons fresh chopped oregano or dill weed

1/2 cups fresh chopped basil

1/4 cup pitted sliced Kalamata olives

1/4 cup feta, crumbled

1/2 cup nonfat ricotta or cottage cheese

1/4 cup grated low-fat mozzarella

3 large egg whites, beaten

1 whole egg, beaten

1 teaspoon nutmeg

1/2 teaspoon black pepper

nonstick spray, or 1 teaspoon olive oil

6 sheets phyllo dough*

* Whole wheat phyllo is available in the freezer section of some health food stores.

Preheat oven to 350 degrees F.

Heat olive oil in a large skillet and sauté onions and garlic until golden, about 5 minutes. Stir in spinach mix, parsley, oregano, and basil, heating until greens wilt slightly. Remove from heat and cool. When room temperature, fold in olives, cheeses, and eggs.

Spray bottom and sides of an 8 x 8 x 2-inch baking dish. Cut phyllo sheets in half. Line the bottom of the dish with a layer of phyllo. Lightly spray or brush with oil. Repeat process with remaining layers. Spread spinach-egg mix evenly over the phyllo and press it into the corners of the pan.

For Topping:

Place a layer of phyllo over spinach mix. Spray with nonstick cooking spray, or brush with olive oil. Repeat process with remaining layers. Press phyllo down into the filling. Curl the edges under.

Bake for 1 hour or until the filling is set and the phyllo delicately browned. Remove from oven and allow 5 minutes for the Spanakopita to rest. Cut into 6 portions and serve hot.

Serving per casserole: 6- to 7-ounce servings	Protein: 12 g	Sodium: 387 mg
Calories per serving: about 195	Fat: 7 g	Potassium: 410 mg
Carbohydrates: 21 g	Fiber: 2.7 g	% Calories from: Carbohydrates: 42%
	Cholesterol: 65 mg	Protein: 24%
		Fat: 34%

Rancho Guacamole

1 cup broccoli florets

1 cup fresh or frozen green peas

6 medium avocados, peeled and seeded

1 cup finely diced tomato

1/2 cup red, yellow, or sweet onion, finely diced

1 green onion, trimmed and thinly sliced

1 jalapeno or serrano pepper, seeded and minced

2 to 3 cloves garlic, minced

1/4 cup chopped fresh cilantro

1/2 teaspoon sea salt, or to taste

4 to 6 tablespoons lime juice

In a saucepan, steam broccoli in a small amount of water until tender. Remove from pan and let cool. Steam the peas in the saucepan with a little water, cooking about 5 minutes. Let vegetables cool.

In a blender or processor, puree vegetable mix until smooth. In a medium-sized bowl mash avocado until creamy. Add in the pureed vegetables, chopped tomato, onions, green onion, pepper, garlic, and cilantro. Season with sea salt and lime juice to taste. Mix well. Transfer to a serving bowl. May be covered tightly and refrigerated for several hours.

Serve with baked yellow corn tortilla wedges* and an array of fresh veggies such as bell pepper strips, jicama, summer squash, and cherry tomatoes.

Yield: About 70 ounces
Calories per ounce: 32 (about 2 tablespoons)
Carbohydrates: 2.2 g
Protein: 0.6 g
Fat: 2.5 g
Fiber: 1.0 g
Cholesterol: 0 mg
Sodium: 15 mg
Potassium: 119 mg
% Calories from: Carbohydrate: 25%
    Protein: 8 %
    Fat: 67%

*Cut tortillas in quarters. Spray bake pan lightly with olive oil. Arrange wedges on pan. Spray wedges lightly with oil and season lightly with sea salt, if desired. Bake in 325 degree F oven until crisp. Four wedges with the oil have about 67.5 calories and 1.7 grams fat.

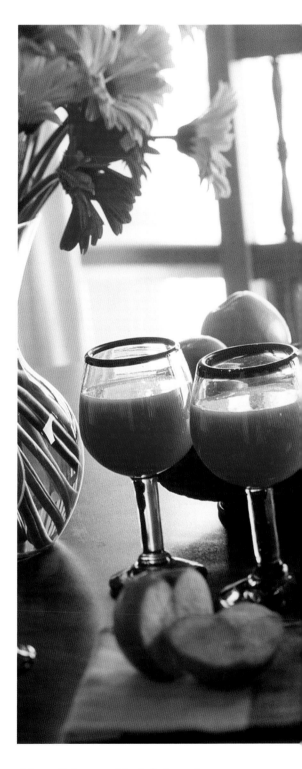

A bountiful array of fresh fruits and juices from Rancho la Puerta's own organic garden, Tres Estrellas. (Courtesy photo)

Candied Ginger Sorbet

1 cup banana, chopped in small cubes
1 cup mango, chopped in small cubes
1 cup pineapple, chopped in small cubes
2 to 3 tablespoons candied ginger, minced
1/2 cup fresh orange juice

Freeze fruit cubes on tray. When solid, remove from freezer and let stand about 5 minutes. Place fruit in a processor cup with the juice and the ginger. Puree until creamy. Serve immediately. Garnish with a sprig of mint and a fresh berry, if desired.

Servings per recipe: 6 3.5-ounce servings
Calories per serving: 78
Carbohydrates: 20 g
Protein: 0.7 g
Fat: 0.2 g
Fiber: 1.5 g

Cholesterol: 0 mg
Sodium: 4 mg
Potassium: 328 mg
% Calories from: Carbohydrates: 94%
    Protein: 3%
    Fat: 4%

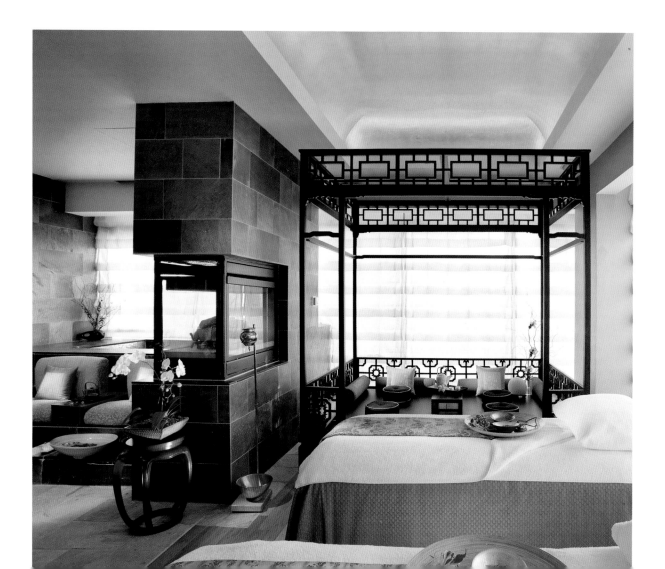

Almond Cookies

1/3 cup unsalted butter

1/2 cup syrup of agave* or maple syrup

2 tablespoons vanilla

1 cup almonds

1 tablespoon ground cinnamon

1/4 cup orange juice

3/4 cup whole wheat pastry flour

Grated rind from 1 whole orange

* This low-glycemic sweetener, indigenous to Meso America, can be found in health food stores.

Preheat oven to 350 degrees F. In a large mixing bowl, cream butter. Add in syrup and vanilla and stir until incorporated. In a blender or processor cup, pulse almonds until a fine meal. Add almonds, cinnamon, juice, flour, and rind to the butter mix. Stir until smooth.

Prepare a baking sheet with nonstick spray. Place two teaspoons of dough side by side on sheet and spread into a thin, elongated form. Repeat process with remaining dough.

Bake at 350 degrees F until golden brown, about 10 minutes.

Servings per recipe: about 43 cookies
Calories per serving: 49
Carbohydrates: 4.7 g
Protein: 0.9 g
Fat: 2.9 g
Fiber: 0.6 g

Cholesterol: 7 mg
Sodium: 0.7 mg
Potassium: 40 mg
% Calories from: Carbohydrates: 37%
Protein: 7%
Fat: 53%

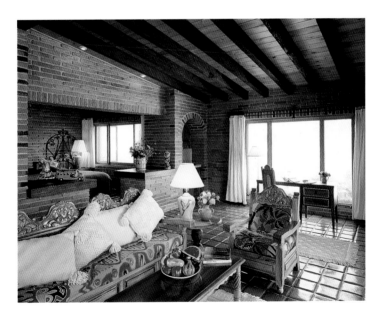

facing: A touch of Chinese imperial splendor in the couples treatment room at New York's Mandarin Oriental Spa. (Courtesy photo)

Tasteful and colorful Mexican furnishings keep spa guests cheerful at Rancho la Puerta. (Courtesy photo)

COOKING TIPS FROM RANCHO LA PUERTA
FITNESS RESORT AND SPA

By Yvonne Nienstadt, Nutrition Director

Look for vibrancy. The most important ingredient in cooking is freshness. Fresh, vibrant natural foods satisfy not only the tongue, but body and brain as well. Choose organic foods whenever possible for their higher nutrient levels and in avoiding toxic chemicals. Nothing tastes like food grown organically and served up within just hours of harvest. Discover your local organic farmers who are participating in a federally funded program for sustainable agriculture called Community Supported Agriculture (CSA). For a CSA farm near you, go to Community Alliance with Family Farmers' Web site, www.caff.org. To find your local farmers' market, visit www.localharvest.org.

Adapt your favorite recipes. This can be done by making them in healthier ways. For example, use whole grain pastas in place of the white flour variety; switch from white rice to brown. Substitute whole wheat pastry flour (made from soft spring wheat) for all or part of the flour called for in cakes or cookies. Avoid commercial white flour, which is not only nutrient deficient, but has been bleached, bromated, and amended with many additives. If your family rebels against whole wheat flour in their favorite treats, use unbleached flour in place of white as it is less processed. For desserts, reduce the quantity of fat and added sweeteners with fruit purees.

Cut the salt. Use fresh or dried herbs and spices, onion, garlic, and shallots to add rich and complex flavors to recipes. Here, south of the border, we are not afraid to use a variety of chiles in our cooking. Dijon and other specialty mustards are wonderful to spark the flavors for sauces and dressings. Rich broths and vegetable purees add tremendous flavor to recipes. Balsamic and flavored vinegars as well as citrus juices can reduce the need for salt in soups and sauces.

Reduce the fat. Use small amounts of cold pressed oils (processed without heat or solvents). These oils are more expensive, but are also more flavorful and healthful. When using oils, try cooking at lower temperatures, rather than frying. This allows foods to braise in their own juices, thus requiring much less fat in cooking. It also keeps the oil from burning. Use nonfat or low-fat cottage cheese or ricotta as a substitute for fatty cheese in recipes. Use aged cheese as a condiment rather than a main ingredient.

Eat more like a vegetarian. Make animal protein the side dish and fill up your plate with lots of salads dressed lightly, steamed or grilled veggies, and a moderate portion of legumes and whole grains. Read Dr. T. Colin Campbell's book *The China Study* for compelling evidence for eating more plant foods, and visit www.thechinastudy.com/.

Keep it simple. Most of us don't have time for hours in the kitchen. Learn to make a few very nutritious meals fast. Have salad fixings and vegetables prepped ahead of time. Make a batch of beans and whole grains that can be used in several dishes a couple of days in a row. Get organized. Once you have a rhythm going, it gets easier. Paulette Mitchell (a regular Rancho presenter) has a wonderful series of cookbooks called *The 15-Minute Gourmet*. Fitness trainer and motivational speaker Rico Caveglia has a good new self-published book, *Real Food Real Fast Lifetime Eating Plan* (http://www.agelesslivinglifestyle.com/).

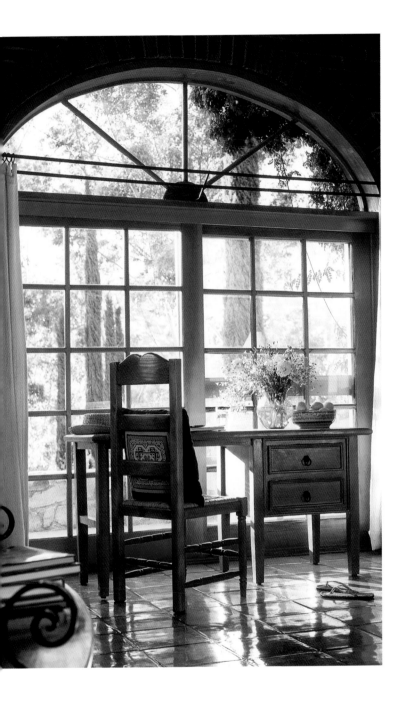

More day spas are also beginning to offer organic foods in their cafés. At BODY Spa & Café[6] in Santa Fe, New Mexico, owner Lorin Parrish boldly states her vision on the menu, right at the very top: "Over 90 percent of our ingredients are organic and we favor locally grown produce." A vegetarian since fifteen, Parrish, who at fifty-five looks twenty years younger and glowing with dynamic vitality, purchases ingredients fresh daily, and those in season (although BODY Café also serves meat dishes).

Having had to battle her own fifteen-year illness after contracting hepatitis and a slew of other pathogens, Parrish turned to India to learn the principles of Ayurvedic cooking as an important part of her self-healing regimen. When she returned to America, she started the New Mexico Healing Academy in 1981.[7]

Parrish opened BODY in summer 2005 to provide various movement classes, to "feed" and transform the body's natural potential to heal with energizing activities, from yoga at different levels (including classes for ages one to three, and on up) to nia (neuromuscular integrative action), created by Debbie and Carlos Rosas in 1983. The Rosas drew their inspiration from nine movement disciplines including dance, Pilates, and the martial arts for fun fitness workouts.[8] Other services like massage and tarot card reading are also on the spa menu at BODY— which makes the Café a bustling social scene all day long until closing time at 9 p.m., every day.

It's easy to kick off your shoes indoors and relax at Rancho la Puerta. (Courtesy photo)

---

[6] BODY Café opens daily at 7 a.m., www.bodyofsantafe.com.

[7] Its Web site, www.nmhealingarts.org, lists cutting-edge classes in various healing modalities, from massage therapy to somatic polarity; the majority of which have their roots in the science of Ayurveda.

[8] The Rosas' book, *The Nia Technique* (Broadway Books, 2005) and www.nia-nia.com are chockfull of lively ideas for this fun dance-Pilates-yoga fusion fitness technique.

Recipes from BODY Café & Spa

All recipes are courtesy of BODY Café, Santa Fe, New Mexico. Created by Lorin Parrish.

BODY Raw Moroccan Soup

Mix the following in food processor until smooth:

2 cups sliced red pepper

2 cups sliced tomato

1 cup sliced zucchini

1 cup purified water

1/4 cup crushed fresh ginger

3/4 cup olive oil

1/2 cup pitted dates

2 teaspoons ground coriander

1 tablespoon ground cumin

1 teaspoon ground cinnamon

1/4 teaspoon cayenne

1 tablespoon Celtic sea salt

Add the following and mix briefly, so pieces of green mint are still visible:

1/2 cup fresh mint leaves

1 tablespoon lemon zest

Remove to a large pot and lightly fold in the following:

1 cup very finely diced red pepper

1 cup finely diced roma tomatoes

To serve: Garnish with chopped mint, organic olive oil, and vinegar.

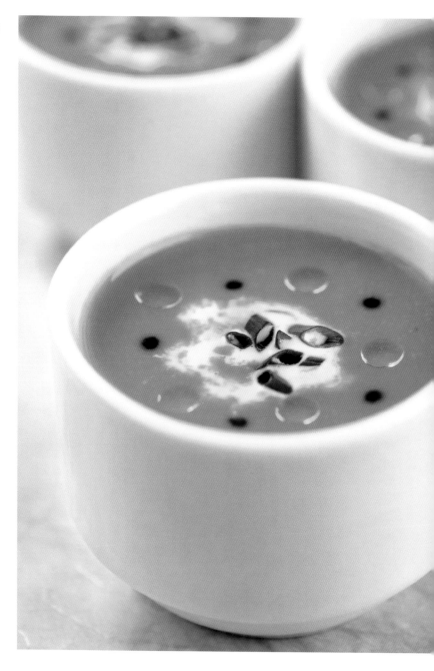

Raw Moroccan Soup, BODY Café & Spa.
(Courtesy photo)

BODY Energy Soup

Carrot mixture:

2 cups filtered water

1 medium carrot, chopped into 1-inch pieces

1 medium apple, chopped

1/2 medium red onion, chopped

1 medium garlic clove, chopped

Place carrot mixture into blender and mix for 30 seconds.

Zucchini mixture:

1 medium zucchini or cucumber, chopped

1 stalk chopped celery

3 to 4 basil leaves

Add zucchini mixture to carrot mixture and blend for another 30 seconds.

Greens:

4 cups loosely packed sprouts, kale, spinach, or baby greens

1 avocado

3 tablespoons organic shoyu (soy sauce)

1/2 teaspoon cumin powder

1 tablespoon Celtic sea salt

Add these green ingredients and blend until creamy.

Add garlic and onion powder to taste.
To serve: Garnish with diced red and yellow peppers, avocado slice, and sunflower sprouts. Yield: 2 quarts

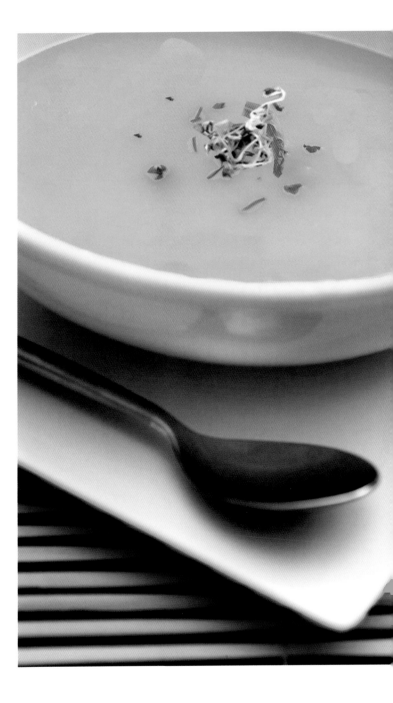

Raw Energy Soup, BODY Café & Spa. (Courtesy photo)

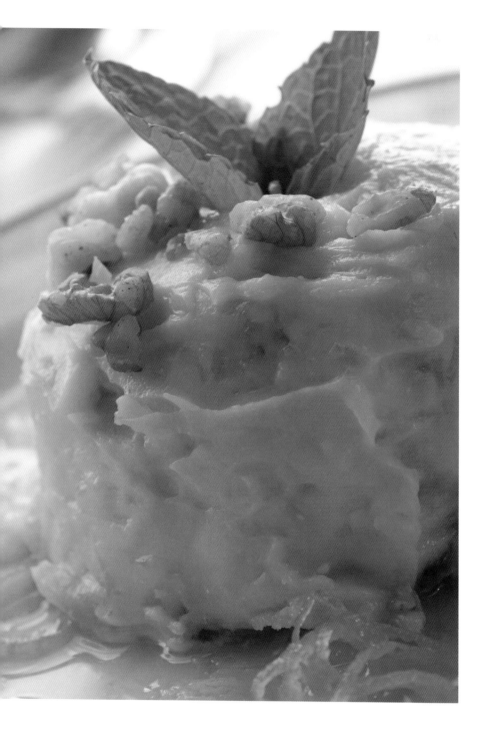

BODY *Banana Chai Smoothie*

3/4 cup organic whole milk
1/2 cup brewed Tazo Chai tea
1 banana
1 cup ice (2 cups for thicker
smoothie)

Puree in blender. Serve with a garnish
of organic whole whipped cream and
cinnamon stick.

BODY *El Favorito (Carrot Juice Cocktail)*

1 3/4 pounds carrots
1 1/2 ounces fresh-squeezed orange juice
1/3 of a medium-sized beet
Ginger (fresh or powdered) to taste

Blend in juicer. Serve chilled with a
garnish of apple or lemon slice.
Makes 1 12-ounce serving.

Raw Carrot Cake, **BODY** Café & Spa.
(Courtesy photo)

BODY Raw Carrot Cake

Carrot Cake Mix

10 cups pureed peeled carrots

2 cups piñon nuts

1/2 cup raisins

1 cup *soaked* dates

water

4 teaspoons pumpkin pie spice

Zest of 2 lemons

2 to 3 tablespoons psyllium seeds (as needed)

Puree carrots and remove. Process piñon, raisins, and dates in blender until creamy. Add water as needed. Mix carrot and piñon mixes together. Add remaining ingredients; set aside.

Carrot Cake Crust

4 cups pureed raisins

2 cups crushed walnuts

Mix thoroughly in food processor.

Coconut Cream Frosting

Flesh of 5 young coconuts

3/4 cup agave nectar

1/4 cup coconut oil

Process all three until smooth and creamy.

Press crust evenly into bottom of cake pan, add half the cake mixture, layer of coconut cream, and add remaining cake mixture; frost top and sides with coconut cream. Garnish with a few carrot shavings, mint sprig, and walnuts. Double Decker Cake. Yields 16 pieces.

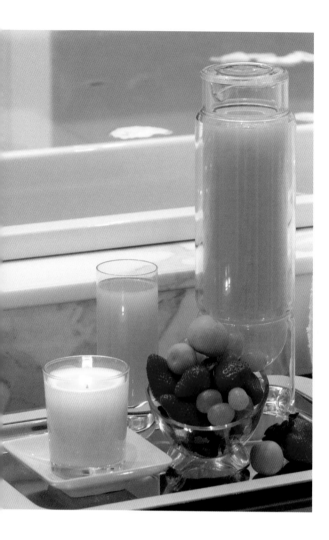

Aesthetician Cornelia Zicu's signature touches at her Cornelia Day Resort & Spa. (Courtesy photo)

facing: Tea time to uplift the senses at Tonia Prestupa's Japanese garden tea-house. Floral arrangement by Mimi Lipps.

Let Thy Food Be Thy Remedy

Novel as the concept of food as medicine may sound today, it is nevertheless as old as the Hippocratic healing precept of "Thy food shall be thy remedy."

Regardless of whether this wisdom is espoused by western-trained physicians such as Henry G. Bieler, Dean Ornish, or Andrew M. Weil (some of their titles are listed in the bibliography at the back) or the Indian science of self-healing, Ayurveda, modern and ancient healers have known all along that nature's pharmacy offers the most effective tools for good health—by healing with herbs and fresh, seasonal foods that complement each person's own unique constitution.

"Experience has taught us that when man becomes burdened with diseases due to acid intoxication, usually from overindulgence of sweets, starches, and proteins, he must turn to the alkaline vegetables for neutralization," writes Dr. Bieler in his book now regarded as a classic in most nutrition schools and classes, *Food Is Your Best Medicine*.[9]

Unlearning old notions to rediscover eating well for one's own unique body cells and tissues takes time. Some years ago, while I was shopping at a Whole Foods Market for organic items, an irate shopper exploded his wrath by loudly accusing the store of overcharging organic foods for economic gain. As for everything, an informed consumer is the best resource to overcoming prejudice and unprogressive ways of thinking—by being personally involved.

The analogy in rediscovering Ayurveda as a self-healing science and other healthy habits (generally acknowledged as folk wisdom) that everyone can benefit from, may take on similar overtones. But time is both a patient friend and an enduring guide—and time will tell. Already, Time is unfolding this rediscovery with exquisite Ayurvedic spa treatments brought up to date by practitioners such as Pratima Raichur (the author of *Absolute Beauty*, mentioned in chapter 3) with her Bindi facial skin-care line used by many spas all across the country.

Respecting food as medicine will, in the long run, enhance a person's immune system by gently assisting the body to fight pathogens naturally, transition healthily with each season's climatic changes, and rebalance the body with nutrients whenever needed.

9 Page 204.

The divine attributes of spa cuisine can easily be enjoyed at home too, as these recipes show. The joy of preparing and eating good food is unparalleled because:

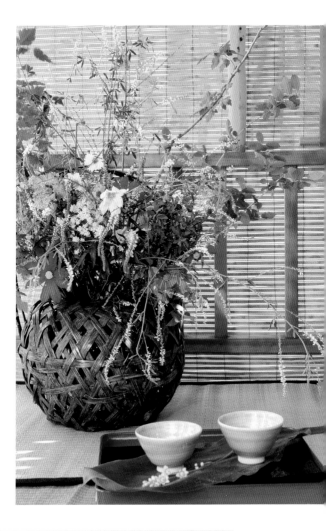

- It enhances the body's immune system in effectively combating pathogens (disease-making organisms that are present everywhere) while bestowing bites of happiness in many delicious ways with one of life's greatest passions.

- Paying a little more at your farmers' market not only turns the sustainable wheels of local sweat and land equity but also puts fresh, seasonal, and organic gifts on your table with pleasant outcomes for everyone. Always ask to buy food that is raised free-range and free of hormones such as BGH (bovine growth hormone).

- By preparing and cooking with a loving consciousness, the cook is able to feed family and friends beyond mere outer eating—as their compassionate emotions also infuse the delectable foods they cook, to bless diners on deeper levels. Diners, in turn, play their part in offering heartfelt gratitude, thus completing the cycle of assimilating on many levels, good food for good health.

DRINKING HABITS TO ENHANCE YOUR IMMUNITY
By Dr. David Frawley, Ayurvedic physician and author

- Avoid drinking ice water before meals, which lowers your body temperature. The body's regular temperature assimilates food intake much more easily, instead of lowering it with ice water.

- Avoid carbonated soft drinks—which have plenty of excess, refined sugars.

- Avoid drinking cold liquids. Instead, drink warm herbal teas and room temperature water, which help your body's metabolism.

Recipes from Ayurvedic Cooking for Self-Healing

Recipes From Ayurvedic Cooking for Self-Healing *by Usha and Vasant Lad. The Ayurvedic Press,* 2002.

Mung Dal Kitchari (Tridoshic)

↓↓↓ The three arrows indicate this recipe balances the three doshas in Ayurvedic nutrition.

1 cup yellow mung dal
1 cup basmati rice
1-inch piece of fresh ginger, peeled and chopped fine
2 tablespoons shredded, unsweetened coconut
1 small handful fresh cilantro leaves
1/2 cup water
3 tablespoons ghee
1 1/2-inch piece of cinnamon bark
5 whole cardamom pods
5 whole cloves
10 black peppercorns
3 bay leaves
1/4 teaspoon turmeric
1/4 teaspoon salt
6 cups water

Wash the mung dal and rice until water is clear. Soaking the dal for a few hours helps with digestibility.

In a blender, put the ginger, coconut, cilantro, and 1/2 cup water and blend until liquefied. Heat a large saucepan on medium heat and add the ghee, cinnamon, cloves, cardamom, peppercorns, and bay leaves. Stir for a moment until fragrant.

Add the blended items to the spices, then the turmeric and salt. Stir until lightly browned.
Stir in the mung dal and rice and mix very well.

Pour in the 6 cups of water, cover and bring to a boil. Let boil for 5 minutes, then turn down the heat to very low and cook, lightly covered, until the dal and rice are soft, about 25 to 30 minutes. Serves 4 to 5.

Kitchari is a cooked mixture of rice, dal, and spices that is easily digested, and high in protein; it complements a mono-fast. This recipe is especially beneficial for tridoshic balancing.

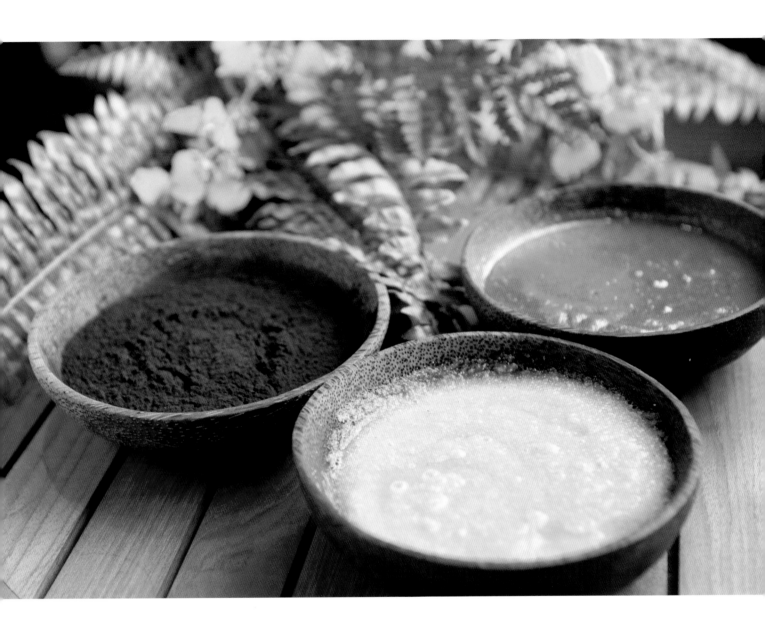

A tempting array of freshly prepared
herbal spa treats at SpaOlakino.
(Courtesy photo)

Mixed Vegetable Subji

↓↓↓   The three arrows indicate this recipe balances the three doshas in Ayurvedic nutrition.

4 cups cut vegetables (green pepper, green beans, zucchini, yellow squash, etc.)

2 tablespoons ghee or safflower oil

1/2 teaspoon cumin seeds

1/2 teaspoon black mustard seeds

1/4 teaspoon ajwan seeds

1/2 teaspoon masala powder or cayenne

1/4 teaspoon turmeric

1 pinch hing

1/4 teaspoon salt

Wash, trim, and cut the vegetables into bite-sized pieces. Try cutting each vegetable into a different shape for a nice visual effect.

Heat a deep frying pan on medium heat and add the oil or ghee, then the cumin seeds, mustard seeds, ajwan, and hing.

When the seeds pop, add the masala or cayenne and turmeric. Stir briefly, then put in the vegetables and salt. Stir to coat them thoroughly with the spices.

Turn down the heat to low and cover. Stir after 5 minutes. Continue cooking on low for another 15 minutes or until the vegetables are just tender. Serves 4.

This subji balances *agni*, or digestive fire, and is laxative. Also good food for bones and joints.

Almond Khir

↓↓↓   The three arrows indicate this recipe balances the three doshas in Ayurvedic nutrition.

1 pinch saffron

40 whole almonds, soaked overnight and peeled

5 cups milk

1/4 teaspoon cardamom

1 rounded teaspoon charole nuts (optional)

1 cup Sucanat or other sugar (or to taste)

1 tablespoon ghee

Soak the saffron in 1 tablespoon warm water for 10 minutes. Put the almonds in a blender with 1 cup of the milk and blend until liquefied. Bring the remaining 4 cups of milk to a boil and add the cardamom, charole nuts, soaked saffron and blended almonds. Stir in the sugar and ghee. Cook for 5 minutes at a gentle boil, stirring occasionally. Serve warm. Serves 4.

Kapha types need to add a pinch of dry ginger and to eat this in moderation.

Chai

↓↓↓   The three arrows indicate this recipe balances the three doshas in Ayurvedic nutrition.

3 cups water

4 cloves

2 pinches ground nutmeg

2 pinches ground cinnamon

2 pinches ground cardamom

1/2-inch piece fresh ginger

1 teaspoon black tea (or dandelion root or lemon grass)

1 cup milk

2 teaspoons sweetener of your choice

Boil the water with the spices for 2 minutes. Add the tea and simmer for 2 minutes. Add the milk and heat until hot but not boiling. Add sweetener and serve. Serves 4.

You may vary the amounts of the milk and sugar according to taste and dosha. Of course, increasing the milk and/or sugar can provoke kapha.

If you use caffeinated tea, the cardamom will help neutralize the effects of the caffeine.

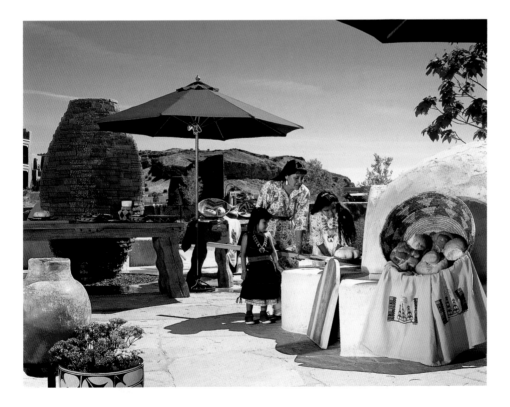

Appreciating Native American culinary arts with the indigenous horno, or beehive-shaped oven, is a creative way to relax and recuperate with family. (Courtesy, Tamaya Mist Spa & Salon)

Recipes from Executive Chef Fabian Valdez

Ojo Caliente Mineral Springs Resort & Spa, Ojo Caliente, New Mexico.

Sopa Azteca

6 pounds chopped tomatoes (tomate machacado works best)

7 1/2-ounce chipotle peppers in adobo

1/2 medium-sized onion, chopped

3 whole fresh garlic cloves

1/4 pound unsalted butter

1 12-inch flour tortilla

Fine grated Monterey jack cheese

Put chopped tomato, chipotle peppers, onion, and garlic in a food processor and puree on high. Remove from food processor and run through a china cap or fine strainer. In a heavy-duty saucepan, place butter and let it melt. When melted, add tomato mixture and bring to a boil; reduce heat and simmer for about 15 minutes. Salt to taste. When done, serve with crispy tortilla strips and grated jack cheese.

Prickly Pear Cactus Flower Vinaigrette

4 sprigs fresh tarragon

1 medium shallot

1 tablespoon Dijon mustard

15 ounces Prickly Pear Cactus puree

3 ounces white wine vinegar

Extra virgin olive oil

1 1/2 ounces granulated sugar

Finely chop tarragon and shallot. Put in food processor; add mustard, cactus puree, and vinegar. Blend on high while adding olive oil. Pour oil as slow as you can—this will help to emulsify it so the vinaigrette will not break (add oil until desired consistency). Add sugar and blend for 30 seconds.

facing: Zen beauty enhances a treatment
room at Ten Thousand Waves Japanese
Spa and Retreat, Santa Fe, New Mexico.

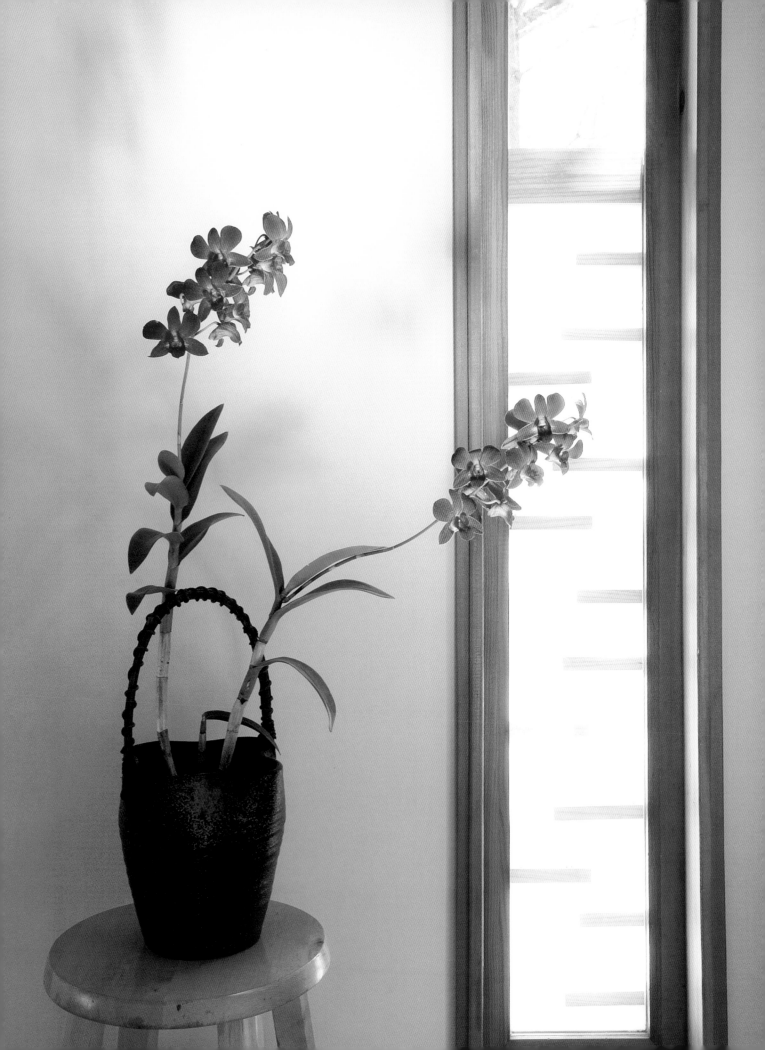

CHAPTER SEVEN

CHOOSING TO GO GREEN

Those of us in the spa industry should be leaders in environmental awareness and action. Without a healthy world, there are no healthy people.[1]

—Deborah Szekely, Founder of Rancho La Puerta Fitness Resort and Spa, Tecate, Mexico

We should all be engaged in conscious actions to preserve our natural assets and scarce resources of the environment.

—Thomas Worrell Jr., Founder of El Monte Sagrado Living Resort & Spa, Taos, New Mexico

Receiving an annual average rainfall of nine to twelve inches, Rancho La Puerta Fitness Resort and Spa is acutely aware of the need to harvest and conserve water—especially crucial in maintaining its mantle of fresh greenery and colorful flora in welcoming 150 weekly guests, year-round. Thanks to Sarah Livia Brightwood's (owner Deborah Szekely's daughter) green thumb and a team of twenty-two full-time gardeners, the Rancho landscape is a serenely captivating canvas anchored by sacred Mount Kuchumaa in the background.

The garden gives the first impression of going green, regardless of the eco-friendly methods used. Rancho's brochure calls itself "probably the world's first 'eco' resort" with its sustainable organic garden (providing luscious fare daily for breakfast and lunch buffets) and innovative resource conservation strategies.

The purpose of this chapter is to move the discussion along for more eco-friendly spas, by recognizing the need to conserve scarce environmental resources given the sizeable commercial operations that spas and resorts are.

Early spring captivates and revives at the entrance to Avanyu Spa at La Posada de Santa Fe.

[1] As reported in the *New York Times*, April 23, 2004, "At Eco-Spas, It's Nature *And* Nurture" by Gretchen Reynolds.

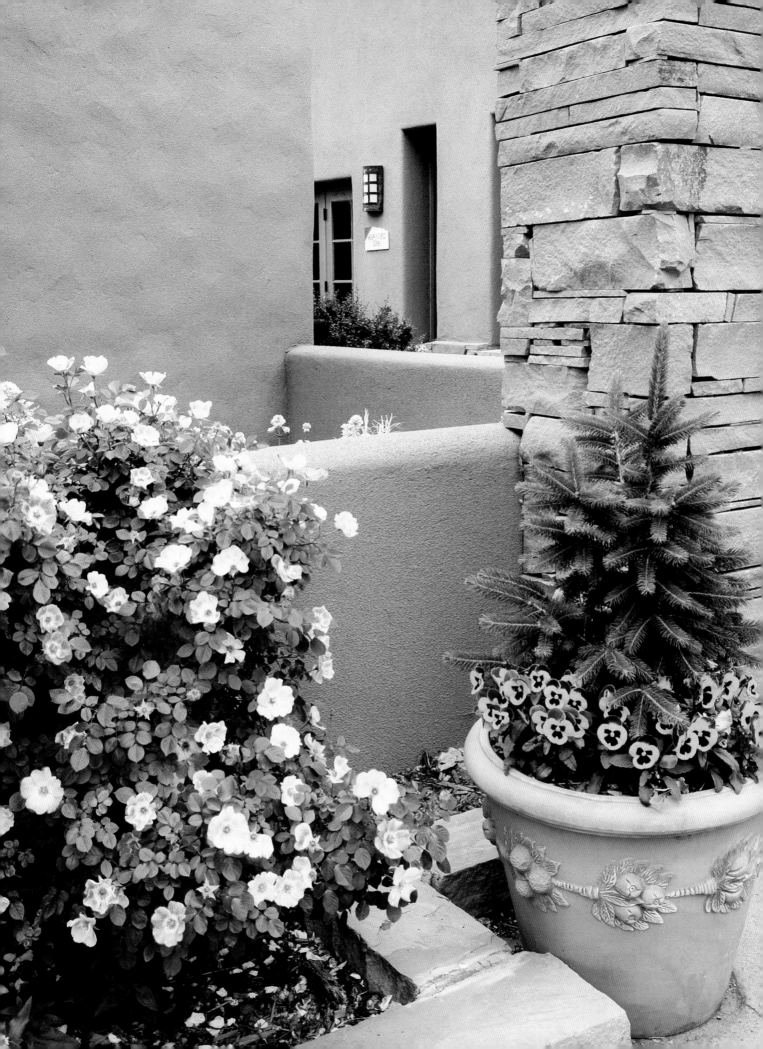

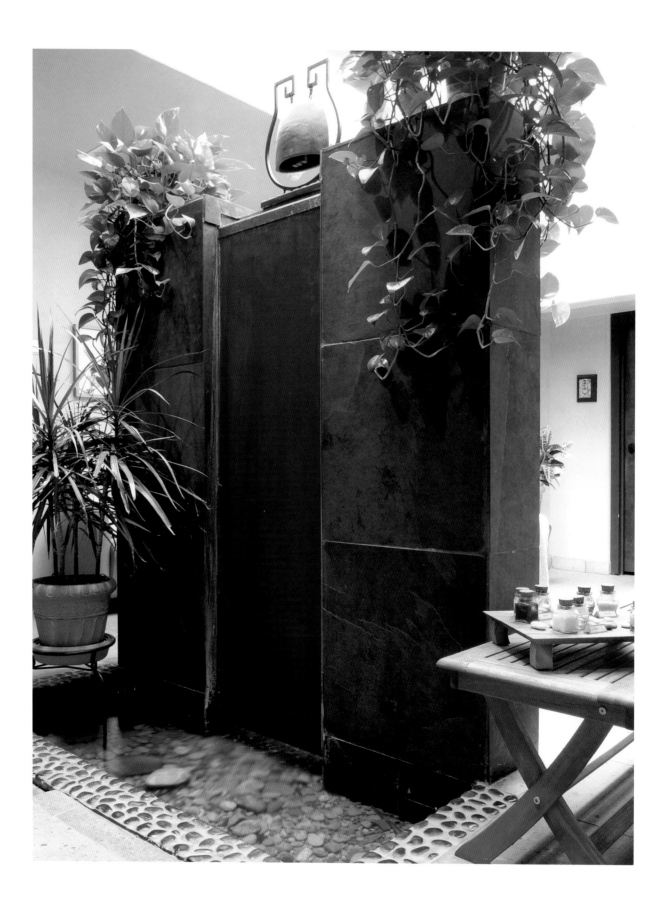

BIODYNAMIC SPA™ DEVELOPMENT

By Eva M. Jensch

A biodynamic spa is a sustainable spa developed to promote sustainability for the planet, people, and profits. Biodynamic spas incorporate product integrity, renewable energy sources, ethical sourcing of resources, cares for health and safety, values its workforce, and includes philanthropic activities and seasonal lifecycles in the development and operation of the spa.

More specifically—

- Works holistically with natural processes and laws of nature to create healthy living environments.
- Creates environments promoting the health of guests and workers.
- Buildings are value-engineered for natural balance, timeless beauty, and functional economy.
- Creates healthy, vital environments that inspire occupants to live healthy lives.
- Utilizes principles that are environmentally sound, socially responsible, and economically feasible.
- Respects an integrated environmental design in honoring site-specific demands and land use.
- Employs healthy building materials and integrative systems with harmonic proportions without altering electromagnetic fields in the area.
- Incorporates living plants, natural light, and natural harvesting water systems to support good health.

facing: The light-filled waiting room at Avanyu Spa at La Posada de Santa Fe captivates with natural textures.

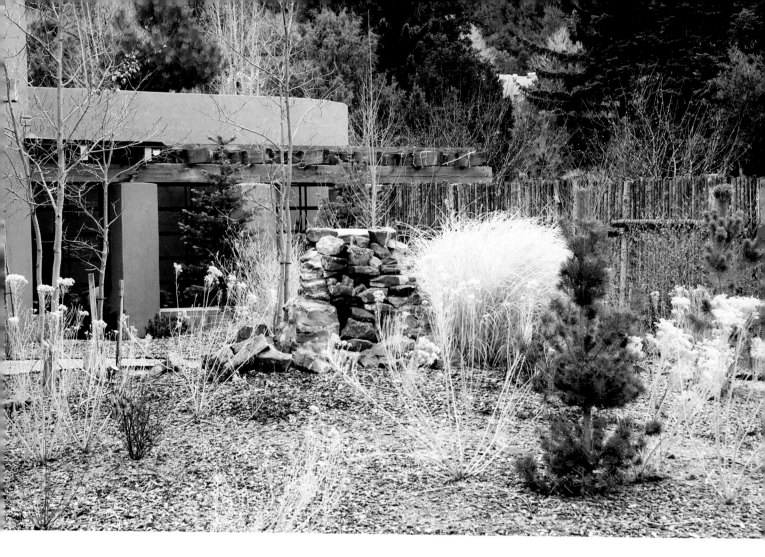

A rustic setting evokes natural serenity for the elegant ShaNah Spa at The Bishop's Lodge north of Santa Fe, New Mexico.

facing: A relaxing outdoor hot tub at Ten Thousand Waves Japanese Spa and Retreat, Santa Fe, New Mexico.

Water Conservation and Landscaping

At the high-desert Absolute Nirvana Spa in Santa Fe, New Mexico, water usage is modest enough that owner Carolyn Lee installed "a UV [ultraviolet] light system that purifies recycled water 99.9 percent; the remaining 0.1 percent waste is easily dissipated by hydrogen peroxide," says Lee. Her state-of-the-art system was designed by Nature's Creations in town, owned by pool-builder Dave Schneider.

Schneider's mega showpiece lies north of Santa Fe, in Taos. Together with then–Dharma Living Systems' owner Thomas Worrell Jr., who designed his (Worrell's) $50 million El Monte Sagrado Living Resort & Spa, Schneider built a "biolarium" based on Worrell's design that recycles gray water (water from sinks). Koi, gold fish, and trout swim in the man-made retention pond that filters black water and aerates it with oxygen to keep bacteria alive. The live bacteria are essential in breaking down nitrites and nitrates in the black water; after this conversion process is through, the water is used for irrigating the gardens.

The high-desert, drought conditions of northern New Mexico encourage another world-renowned spa, Ojo Caliente, to create its

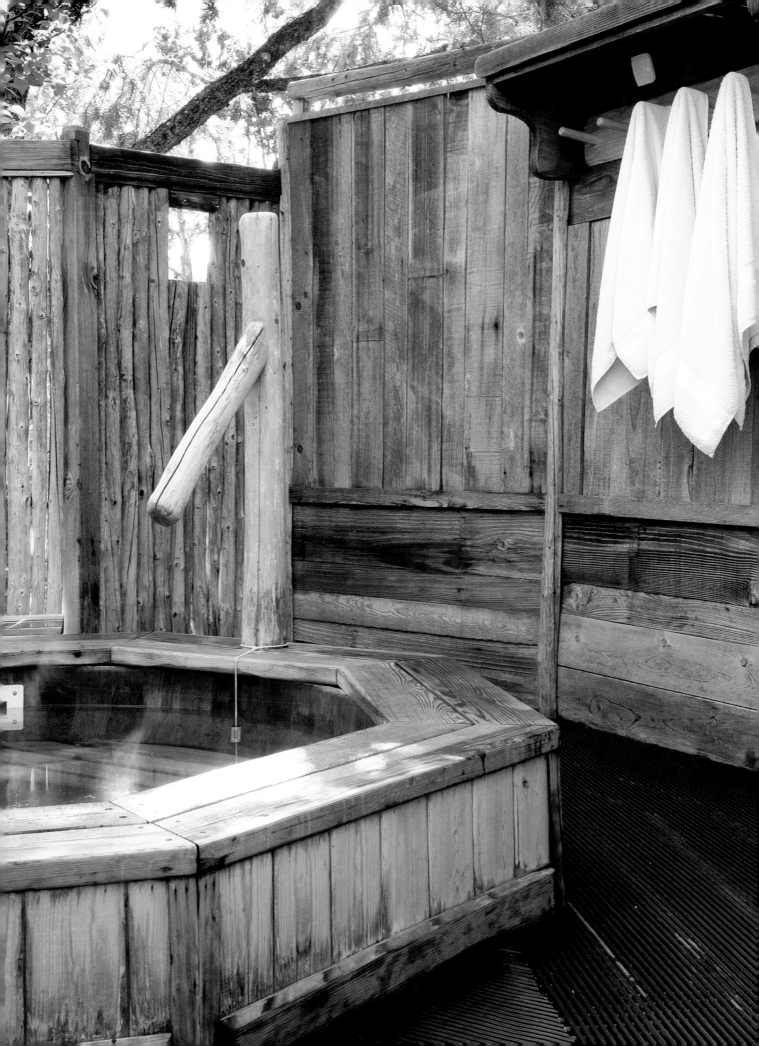

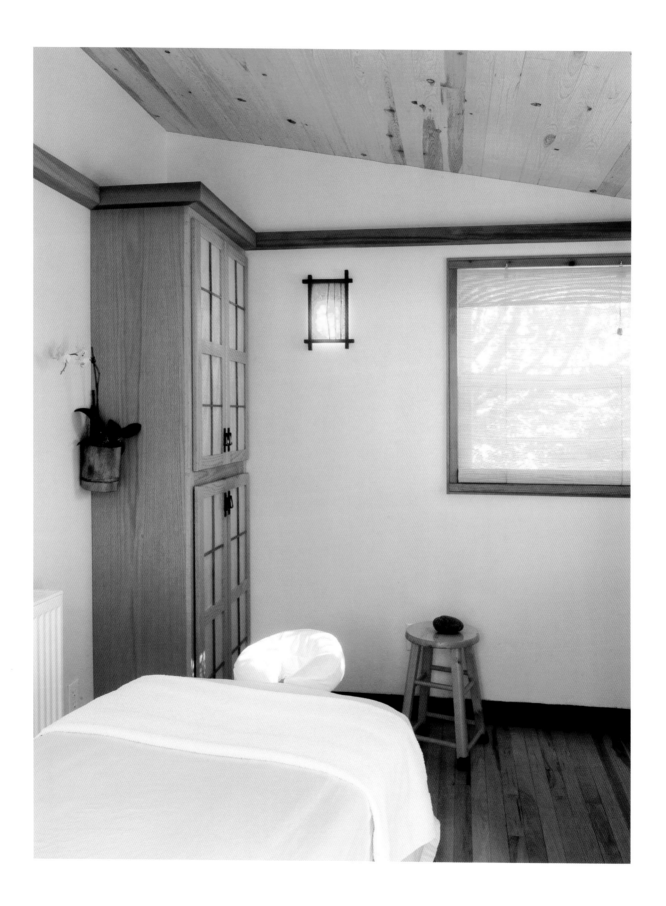

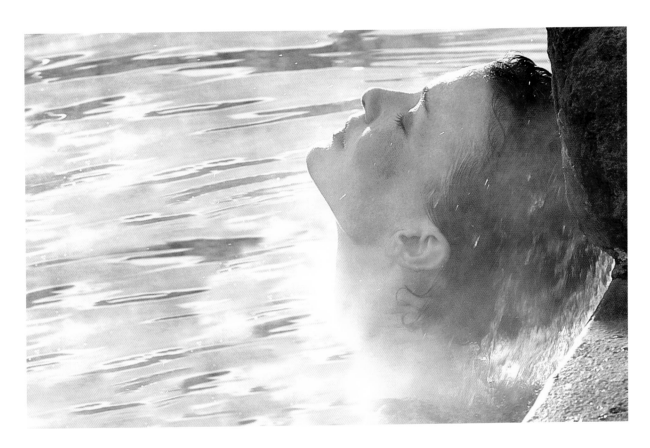

own state-of-the-art systems, as well. John Young, facility manager at Ojo Caliente, says, "The original Indian settlers, ancestors of today's Tewa tribes, were skilled masters of water flow. They designed berms for water catchment away from dwellings and used stones for mulching to prevent water evaporation." Young uses conch shells for mulching from a Las Cruces in-state company.

Energy Consumption

The crowning glory of Ojo Caliente's conservation efforts is the radiant heating and cooling system being designed to harness its hot springs' geothermal potential. John Young estimates yearly savings of about 30 percent in weaning away from propane gas that the spa now uses for energy purposes, and decreasing CFCs (chloroflorocarbons) that propane emits in depleting Earth's protective ozone layer.

At Rancho La Puerta, compact fluorescent lighting, which uses less energy, has replaced incandescent bulbs, and although the initial cost of the bulbs was high, savings are realized over the years. Tubular skylights funnel in natural light for guest rooms, gyms, and spa facilities.

facing: Touches of Zen serenity in a treatment room at Ten Thousand Waves Japanese Spa and Retreat, Santa Fe, New Mexico.

Head to head with healing waters at Ojo Caliente, New Mexico. (Courtesy photo)

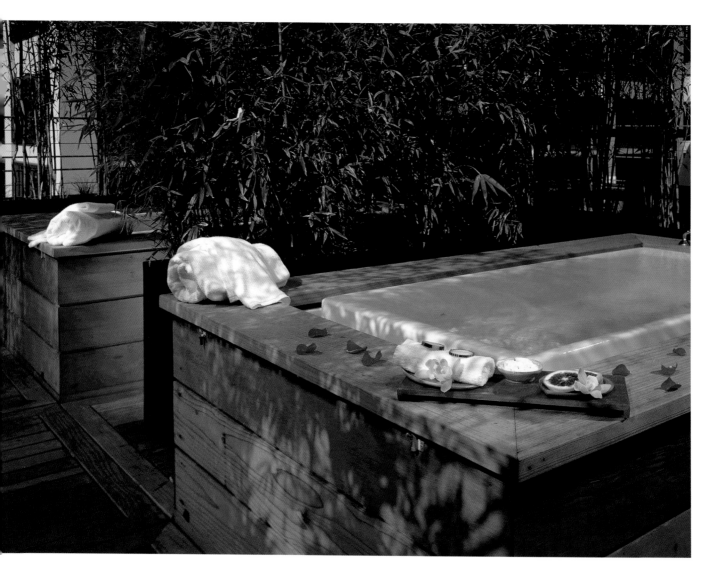

Spa Vitale's rooftop baths are screened from San Francisco's high-rise buildings by bamboo fronds. (Courtesy photo)

facing: The communal coldwater dip refreshes between takes of hot tubbing and sauna at Ten Thousand Waves Japanese Spa and Retreat, Santa Fe, New Mexico.

Waste Treatment

Not many spas have installed composting toilets as Rancho has, while its non-composting toilets in guest rooms and casitas are all low-flow to reduce water consumption. Rancho's on-site waste treatment facility filters gray water for the drip system that irrigates the colorful floral and verdant landscape—looking even more jewel-like in the arid setting.

Ojo has a local waste treatment facility that treats about 250,000 gallons monthly, in allowing clean water to seep back to the local aquifer, which in turn supplies well water for the local community. The layers of geological formations in the area naturally filter and recycle water that percolates through, from rainwater to treated water.

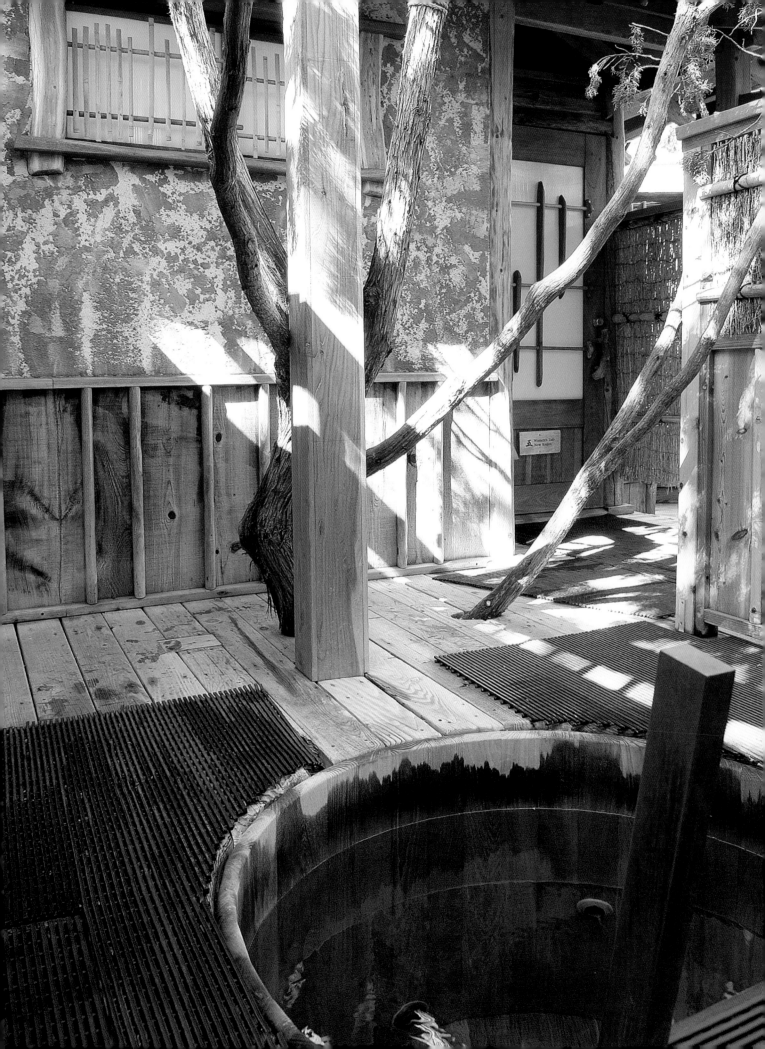

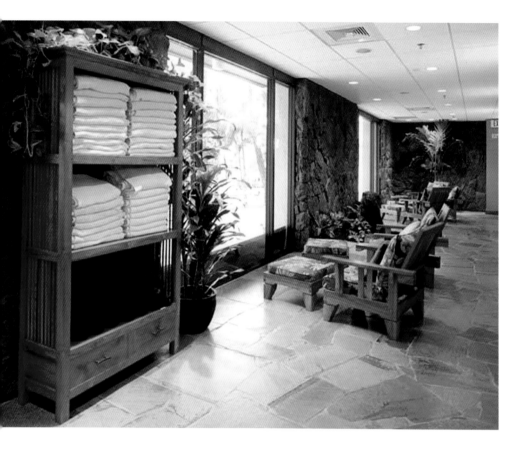

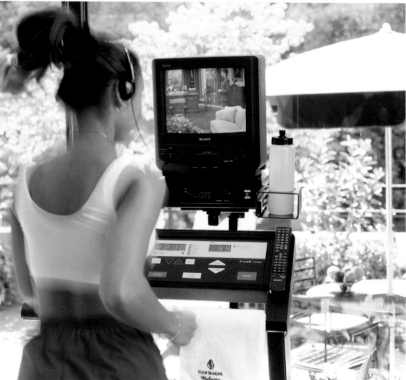

Construction, Conservation, and Building Materials

One conservation effort impacting the local economy is Ojo's purchasing native wood products for new construction. John Young buys from local supplier Lou Salazar (owner of Salazar Enterprises), who salvages wood from areas burnt down by forest fires in Taos County and other surrounding areas.

To avoid landfill pollution and bypass dumping fees, Young donates reusable items to the local fire department and the Habitat for Humanity's ReStore in Espanola, twenty miles away. His reason? "Whatever we cannot find a use for, someone else will," Young states. "This way, we're all actively engaged in reusing, recycling, and finding renewable ways to sustain the environment."

In the town of Taos, an hour's drive away, El Monte Sagrado Living Resort & Spa was an old motor lodge, until present owner Tom Worrell bought it and restored it to a five-star eco-luxury resort. "We should all be engaged in conscious actions to preserve our natural assets and scarce resources of the environment," Worrell advocates. In walking the talk, Worrell has also been instrumental in buying up and rehabilitating many old buildings in town.

Armed with his vision of "the trickle down effect," Worrell aimed to show-and-tell guests (who are typically more affluent decision-makers and visionaries in their own professional fields) how eco-sustainability works for mega resorts, which impacts the environment more intensely.

"El Monte, which opened in June 2003, has been a catalyst in redefining eco-tourism for the spa industry," says Doug Patterson, LEED certified architect and co-owner of the previous Dharma Living Systems, now renamed Living Designs Group. "It used to be eco-tourism meant trekking to a remote retreat to renew and to revive, but now, eco-resorts and spas practice responsibly sustainable strategies," Patterson explains.

Patterson cites two luxury eco-resorts drawing inspiration from El Monte—Sun Palace by Shadows Ranch, an hour's drive west of Denver, Colorado, set to open in 2008, and a yet-unnamed resort north of Georgia in the Blue Mountains, an hour-and-half drive north of Atlanta.

And the Facts Are . . .

"Three out of four Americans think their life is out of balance, and one out of three is looking to do something about it," says Kevin Kelly, president of Canyon Ranch Spa in Arizona.[2] Kelly believes that by 2025, half of the U.S. population "will be actively pursuing a way to live greener, healthier, and more psychologically satisfying lives."

Canyon Ranch Spa's research predicts "the emergence of a $400 billion to $1 trillion market in 'wellness lifestyles' consisting of the health, beauty, food, fitness, medicine, spirituality, and of course, spa industries," a *New York Times* article reported.

Inevitably, a person has to want to live a balanced, healthy life. "Sustainability starts with us. In sustaining the body's good health, we may prevent health issues from escalating," says Sierra Vorel, spa director of El Monte Sagrado Living Resort & Spa.

El Monte Sagrado is Spanish for sacred mountain—and a symbol of divine protection for the sacred resources of Mother Earth. Mount Kuchumaa also is a sacred mountain guiding the eco-sustainability of Rancho La Puerta Fitness Resort and Spa since 1940.

facing, top: Volcanic rock walls add arresting textures to the waiting room at SpaOlakino, Honolulu. (Courtesy photo)

facing, bottom: Dynamic movement works its magic in rejuvenating oxygen cells for instant energy.

[2] Reported by Philip Nobel in "Living In Zen: The Spa Life, 24/7," *New York Times*, November 2, 2006.

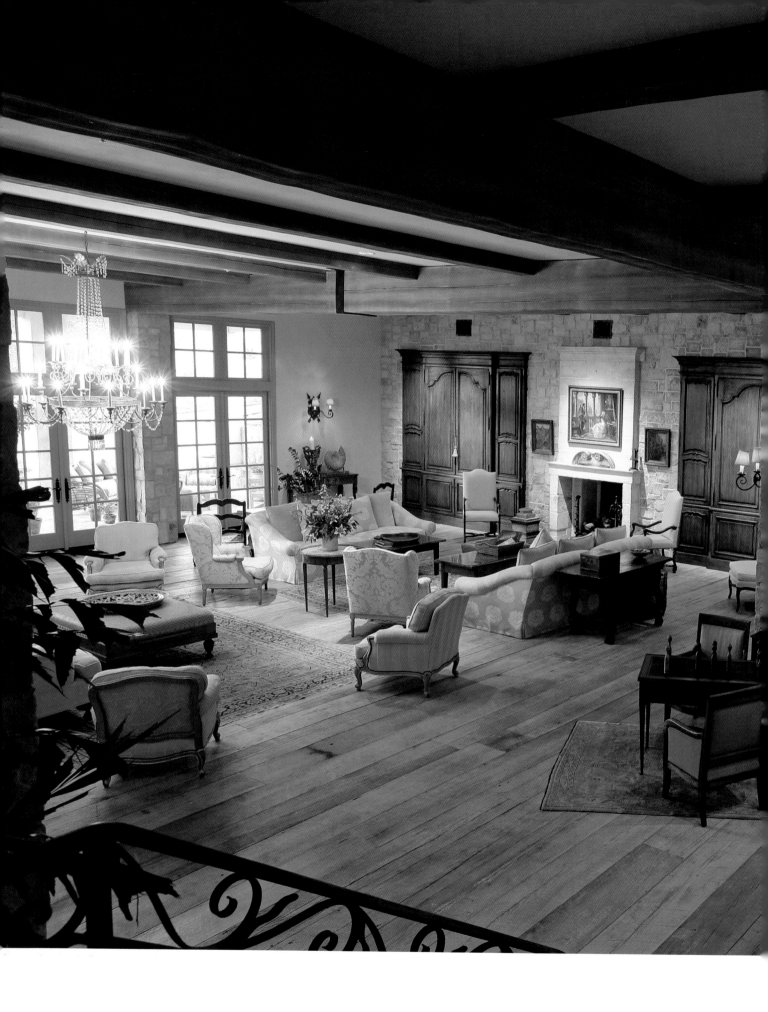

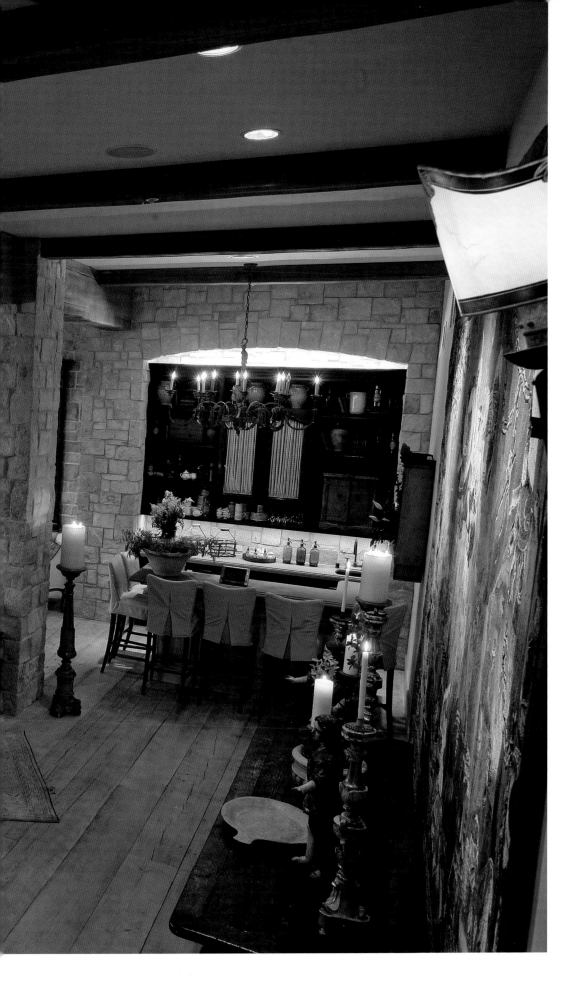

French country
elegance with one-of-
a-kind antiques
transports spa guests
at Cal-a-Vie.
(Courtesy photo)

RESOURCES

DAY SPAS & RESORTS

Absolute Nirvana Spa
106 Faithway Street
Santa Fe, New Mexico 87501
Tel: 505-983-7942
www.absolutenirvana.com

Avanyu Spa at La Posada de
Santa Fe Resort & Spa
330 East Palace Avenue
Santa Fe, New Mexico 87501
Tel: 505-986-0000
www.rockresorts.com

BODY Spa & Café
333 Cordova Road
Santa Fe, New Mexico 87505
Tel: 505-986-0362
www.bodyofsantafe.com

Chopra Center & Spa at Dream
1710 Broadway
New York, New York 10019
Tel: 212-246-7600
www.chopracenterny.com

Cornelia Day Spa & Resort
663 5th Avenue (between 52nd &
53rd streets)
New York, New York 10022
Tel: 212-871-3050
www.cornelia.com

El Monte Sagrado Living Resort & Spa
317 Kit Carson Road
Taos, New Mexico 87571
Tel: 800-828-TAOS
www.elmontesagrado.com

Four Seasons Hotel New York
57 East 57th Street
(between Park & Madison)
New York, New York 10022
Tel: 212-758-5700
www.fourseasons.com/newyorkfs/

The Spa at Four Seasons Hotel
Philadelphia
One Logan Square
Philadelphia, Pennsylvania 19103
Tel: 215-405-2815
www.fourseasons.com/philadelphia

The Spa at Four Seasons Hotel
Washington, D.C.
2800 Pennsylvania Avenue NW
Washington, D.C. 20007
Tel: 202-324-0444
www.fourseasons.com/washington

God's Beauty Skin Care
84–47 164th Street
Jamaica, New York 11432
Tel: 718-526-2954

Ihilani Resort & Spa
Ko Olina Resort
92–1001 Olani Street
Kapolei, Hawaii 96707
Tel: 808-679-0079
www.ihilani.com

Mandarin Oriental, The Spa at
80 Columbus Circle at 60th Street
New York, New York 10023
Tel: 212-805-8880
www.mandarinoriental.com

Mandarin Oriental
1330 Maryland Avenue SW
Washington, D.C. 20024
Tel: 202-787-6100
www.mandarinoriental.com

Nidah Spa at Eldorado Hotel
309 West San Francisco
Santa Fe, New Mexico 87501
Tel: 505-995-4535
www.NidahSpa.com

Nob Hill Spa at The Huntington
1075 California Street
San Francisco, California 94108
Tel: 415-345-2888
www.huntingtonhotel.com

The entrance to the Palm Springs Parker
Meridien Spa in California. (Courtesy photo)

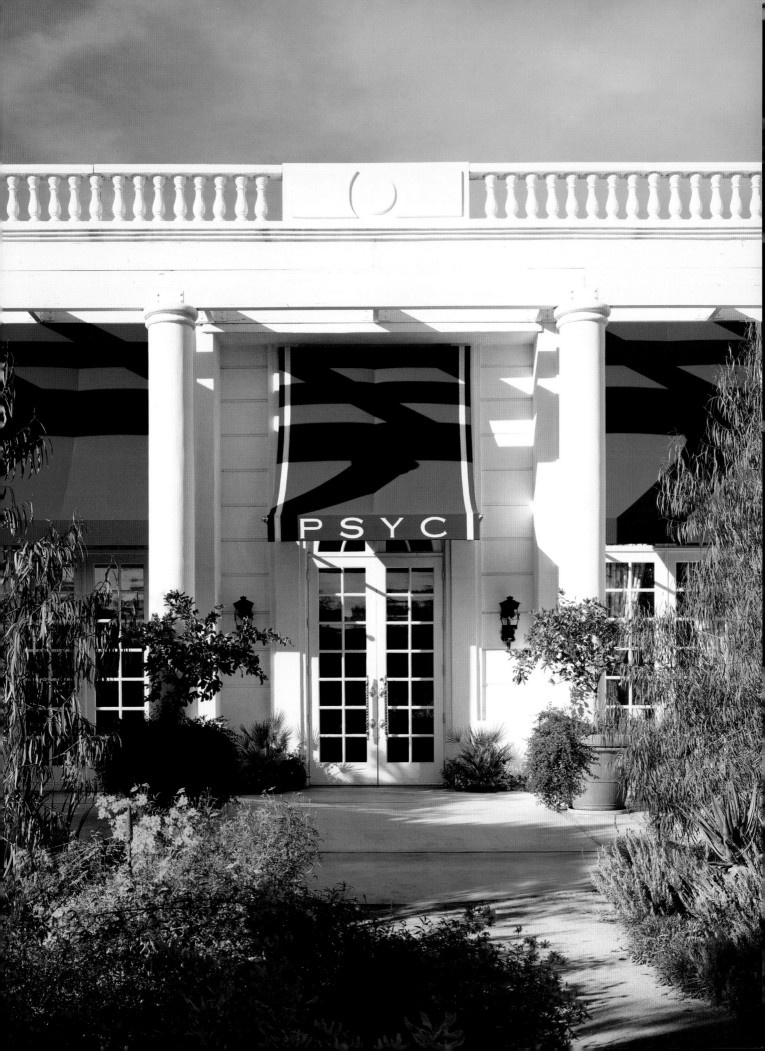

Ojo Caliente Spa (mineral springs)
50 Los Banos Drive
Ojo Caliente, New Mexico 87549
Tel: 800-222-9162
www.ojocalientespa.com

Olympus Spa (Korean)
(1) 3815 196th Street SW Suite160
Lynnwood, Washington 98036
Tel: 425-697-3000
(2) 8615 S. Tacoma Way
Lakewood, Washington 98499
Tel: 253-588-3355
www.olympusspa.com

Gravity Fitness and Spa at
Parker Meridien New York
119 West 56th
(between 6th and 7th avenues)
New York, New York 10019
Tel: 212-708-7340
www.parkermeridien.com

Parker Meridien Palm Springs
4200 East Palm Canyon Drive
Palm Springs, California 92264
Tel: 760-770-5000
www.theparkerpalmsprings.com

Pratima Ayurvedic Skin Care
110 Greene Street, Suite 701
New York, New York 10012
Tel: 212-581-8136
www.pratimaskincare.com

Ritz-Carlton Spa, The
50 Central Park South, 2nd Floor
New York, New York 10019
Tel: 212-521-6135
www.ritzcarlton.com

Safety Harbor Resort & Spa
105 N. Bayshore Drive
Safety Harbor, Florida 34695
Tel: 888-237-8772
www.safetyharborspa.com

Salish Lodge & Spa
P.O. Box 1109
Snoqualmie, Washington 98065
Tel: 800-272-5474
www.salishlodge.com

ShaNah Spa
Bishop's Lodge Resort & Spa
P.O. Box 2367
Santa Fe, New Mexico 87504
Tel: 800-974-2624
www.bishopslodge.com

SpaHalekulani
2199 Kalia Road
Honolulu, Hawaii 96815
Tel: 808-931-5322
www.halekulani.com

SpaOlakino
2552 Kalakaua Avenue
Honolulu, Hawaii 96815
www.spaolakino.com

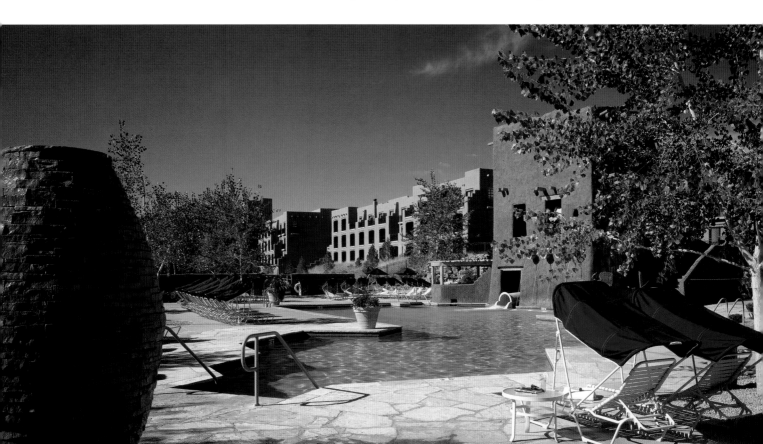

SpaTerre at Inn & Spa at Loretto
Old Santa Fe Trail and Alameda
Santa Fe, New Mexico 87501
Tel: 505-984-7997
www.innatloretto.com

Spa Vitale
8 Mission Street
San Francisco, California 94105
Tel: 415-278-3788
www.spavitale.com

Sunrise Springs Spa Samadhi
242 Los Pinos Road
Santa Fe, New Mexico 87507
Tel: 800-955-0028
www.sunrisepsprings.com

Tamaya Mist Spa & Salon
Hyatt Regency Tamaya Resort & Spa
1300 Tuyuna Trail
Santa Ana Pueblo, New Mexico
    87004
Tel: 505-771-6134
www.tamaya.hyatt.com

Ten Thousand Waves Japanese Spa
& Resort
3451 Hyde Park Road
Santa Fe, New Mexico 87501
Tel: 505-992-5025
www.tenthousandwavs.com

Terme Di Aroma
32 North Third Street
Philadelphia, Pennsylvania 19106
Tel: 215-829-9769
www.termediaroma.com

The Westin New York at Times Square
270 West 43rd Street
New York, New York 10036
Tel: 888-627-7149
www.westinnewyork.com

DESTINATION SPAS

The Ayurvedic Institute (Indian)
Panchakarma Program
11311 Menaul Boulevard N.E.
Albuquerque, New Mexico 87112
Tel: 505-291-9698
www.ayurveda.com

Cal-a-Vie
29402 Spa Havens Way
Vista, California 92084
Tel: 866-772-4283
www.calavie.com

Golden Door®
P.O. Box 463060
Escondido, California 92046
Tel: 800-424-0777
www.goldendoor.com

Miraval Resort & Spa
5000 E. Via Estancia Miraval
Catalina, Arizona 85739
Tel: 800-825-4000
www.miravalresort.com

Rancho La Puerta
P.O. Box 463057
Escondido, California 92046
Tel: 800-443-7565
www.rancholapuerta.com

SKIN CARE PRODUCTS

Benedetta Aromatherapeutics
P.O. Box 5405
Petaluma, California 94055
Tel: 888-868-8331
www.benedetta.com

Bindi Facial Skin Care
P.O. Box 750-250
Forest Hills, New York 11375
Tel: 800-952-4634
www.bindi.com

derma e® Natural Bodycare
4485 Runway Street
Simi Valley, California 93063
Tel: 800-521-3342
www.dermae.net

Desert Blends of Taos
P.O. Box 2126
Rancho de Taos, New Mexico
    87557
Tel: 505-758-4000
www.desertblends.com

Dr. Hauschka Skin Care, Inc.
59 North Street
Hatfield, Massachusetts 01038
Tel: 800-247-9907
www.drhauschka.com

Golden Door Skin Care
P.O. Box 463060
Escondido, California 92046
Tel: 800-231-1444
www.goldendoorskincare.com

facing: Getting away to clear, blue skies and taking to the water
is salubrious and healing. (Courtesy, Tamaya Mist Spa & Salon)

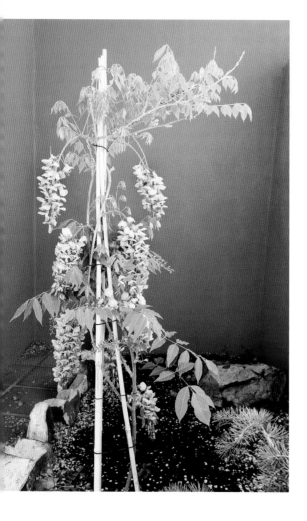

Wisteria against Spa Smadhi's adobe wall celebrates spring at Sunrise Springs, Santa Fe.

Jurlique Holistic Skin Care, Inc.
11 East 44th Street, 8th Floor
New York, New York 10017
Tel: 800-854-1110
www.jurlique.com

JURLIQUE of Santa Fe
De Vargas Center
179C Paseo De Peralta
Santa Fe, New Mexico 87501
Tel: 888-558-7545; 505-982-5125

El Milagro Herbs
Herbalist Tomas Enos, PhD
1020 Canyon Road
Santa Fe, New Mexico 87501
Tel: 505-820-6321
www.milagro-herbs.com

MyChelle Dermaceuticals, LLC
P.O. Box 70
Frisco, Colorado 80443
Tel: 800-447-2076
www.mychelleusa.com

N. V. Perricone Flagship Store
791 Madison Avenue
New York, New York 10021
Tel: 866-791-7911
www.nvperriconemd.com

Weleda
www.usa.weleda.com

MISCELLANY
Caldrea
Natural household cleaning products
Tel: 877-576-8808
www.caldrea.com

Fresh Wave®
Eliminates odors with earth-friendly products
Tel: 800-662-6367
www.fresh-wave.com

Living Designs Group
LEED certified architects
125 La Posta Road, Suite A
Taos, New Mexico 87571
Tel: 505-751-9481
www.livingdesignsgroup.com

Mrs. Meyers
Natural household cleaning products
Tel: 877-865-1508
www.mrsmeyers.com

Naturopatch™ of Vermont
Essential oil body patches
www.naturopatch.com

New Mexico Academy of Healing Arts
501 Franklin Avenue
Santa Fe, New Mexico 87501
Tel: 888-808-5188; 505-982-6271
www.nmhealingarts.org

Resting in the River
Organic biodynamic products
www.restingintheriver.com

Spa Concepts International
Biodynamic Spa™ design concepts
21548 Hyde Road
Sonoma, California 95476
Tel: 707-939-0101
www.spaconcepts.com

GLOSSARY OF SPA TERMS

Acupuncture: The centuries-old Chinese method of healing by inserting sterilized needles at various points of the body to correct and realign energy flow.

Acupressure: Applying pressure on vital areas of the body to correct its energy flow.

Alkaline-Acid Balance: The body's homeostasis for balanced bodily functions, depending on how alkaline or acid it is. The most critical pH balance (or potential for Hydrogen) is in the blood—between the narrow reading of 7.35 and 7.45. The body will extract whatever it needs from bones and tissues to maintain this strict pH range.

Alkaline foods are preferred over acidic because body cells constantly excrete acidic wastes after the body's 75 trillion cells metabolize or extract energy from food intake. Serious consequences also ensue when lifestyle factors (stress, smoking, and pollution, among others) contribute to acidity.

Ranging from 0 to 14, 7.0 is neutral, with lower numbers indicating acidity and higher numbers alkalinity. The preferred food intake ratio is 80:20, of alkaline to acid foods. The pH reading for skin and hair is typically 5.0.

Aromatherapy: The use of natural, essential oils in candles, incense, and spray mists to clear the air and refresh the senses.

Ayurveda: Meaning "the science of life" in Sanskrit, and integrating body-mind-soul wellness, *Ayurveda* is a wellspring of over five thousand years of holistic self-healing wisdom culled from India's sacred health sciences. *Ayurveda* has influenced many western healing modalities such as homeopathy, aromatherapy, psychiatry, nutrition, and polarity therapies.

Biodynamics: An ecologically correct farming approach to sustaining the land organically and in harmony with the seasons promulgated by the German scientist Rudolf Steiner in 1924. Even then, Steiner was concerned about the use of chemical fertilizers and pesticides and the spiritual loss of considering the environment's integrity.

Chi Nei Tsang: A Chinese massage technique called "beautification of the navel" in re-aligning the body's meridians for unobstructed energy flow, as anchored by the navel.

Collagen: An important protein-based body tissue that strengthens blood vessels; makes skin look young with vibrant energy; reduces wrinkling and therefore, the appearance of aging; and is a major component of cartilage, teeth, and bones, as well.

Day spa: A location to receive services that may take from half an hour to a few hours to complete, such as a manicure, facial, or body massage.

Destination spa: A location where guests stay from three to seven days in peaceful, upscale surroundings. Daily, planned activities promote healthy lifestyle changes—from encouraging weight loss or gain, to various aerobic and anaerobic exercises, to healing modalities, to awakening spiritual insights for self-improvement with meditation.

Detoxify: Getting rid of bodily wastes through sweating, naturally occurring metabolic effluents of body cell metabolism, and emotional stress. The process of elimination is as important as ingestion for the body to maintain optimal health.

Dosha: In *Ayurveda*, the *dosha* indicates the body's constitutional energy or how a person's synergy of mind-body activities affects total health. *Doshas* consist of: *vata* (affecting movement), *pitta* (digestion and metabolism), and *kapha* (lubrication) energies, which balance out the person for a sense of total well-being. When imbalance occurs, food combinations relevant to the person's *dosha(s)* help rebalance the body, as do exercise, rest, and meditation.

Essential oils: Natural distillations of essences of herbs, spices, and flowers used for oils and waters, without using petrochemical imitations harmful to skin and body.

Exfoliation: The gentle removal of dead skin cells for new cells to grow. New cells add a natural sheen and vibrancy to the skin, while dead skin cells make it look lifeless.

FIR (Far Infrared Rays): Discovered by German scientist Friedrich Wilhelm Herschel in spring 1800, these energy wavelengths penetrate the skin deeply, unlike solar rays that burn the skin. FIR energy helps stabilize the body's circulatory systems, normalizes blood pressure, activates collagen production essential for healthy skin and bodily functions, and delights weight-loss patients by breaking down fat cells.

Furo: A traditional Japanese bathtub.

Going green: The conscious act of respecting nature's limited resources such as water and clean air to promote a healthy living environment for people, plants, and the land.

Homeopathy: The application of highly diluted doses mimicking a person's symptoms, as in treating like with like, introduced by German physician Samuel Hahnemann in 1807.

Hydrosols: By-products of the steam distillation of essential oils, and less costly than essential oils.

Ingrown hair: Hair follicles that cannot penetrate the thick outer skin or dermis, resulting in a painful ingrown condition with hair growing back down to, and irritating, the dermis.

Lomi lomi: A Hawaiian deep massage technique to detoxify and relax the body.

Lulur: The seventeenth-century Javanese technique of exfoliating the skin with spices and herbs for brides-to-be, now adapted by modern spas for a touch of the exotic.

Metabolism: The body's neuro-chemical cellular processes extracting nutrients from food intake and eliminating wastes and by-products. This exchange fuels the body's energy requirements by constantly recharging it with new energy and a zest for living.

Ohn-dol-bang: A Korean bathhouse and spa.

Onsen: Japanese mineral springs (over 2,500 in Japan) providing natural relaxation, while their curative qualities are taken for preventive health measures, as well.

Pathogens: Disease-causing organisms that are very much a part of the ecosystem. Strengthening the body's immune system goes a long way to fending off afflictions that could deteriorate into disease.

pH: The "potential of Hydrogen" as discussed above in the Alkaline-Acid Balance definition, in contributing to homeostasis or balanced bodily functions.

facing: **An exotic landscape rings the Palm Springs Parker Meridien Spa in California. (Courtesy photo)**

Reflexology: Pin-pointing areas of the sole of the foot related to various parts of the body and applying pressure to unclog energy lines in rebalancing a person's energy.

Sauna: Developed by the Finnish to enhance the body's immune system, the sauna enables a person to sweat out toxins in a hot, dry, cedar-lined room heated to over 100 degrees Celsius.

Scrubs: In body scrubs, the body skin is gently exfoliated with a soft brush, and then rehydrated with natural oils, allowing new skin cells to regenerate healthily.

Sento: A Japanese public bath.

Shiatsu: A Japanese deep-tissue massage that mitigates aches, pains, and stress.

Spa: From the Latin, *sanus per aquum*, or health through water.

Terme: The Italian term for taking to the waters for good health.

Thai massage: A unique dry body massage from Thailand, done with the clothing on.

Thalassotherapy: A Greek water therapy utilizing filtered sea water.

Watsu: A Japanese water therapy administered by a therapist in a pool to reduce a patient's aches and joint pain.

Yasuragi: A Japanese-style head and neck massage.

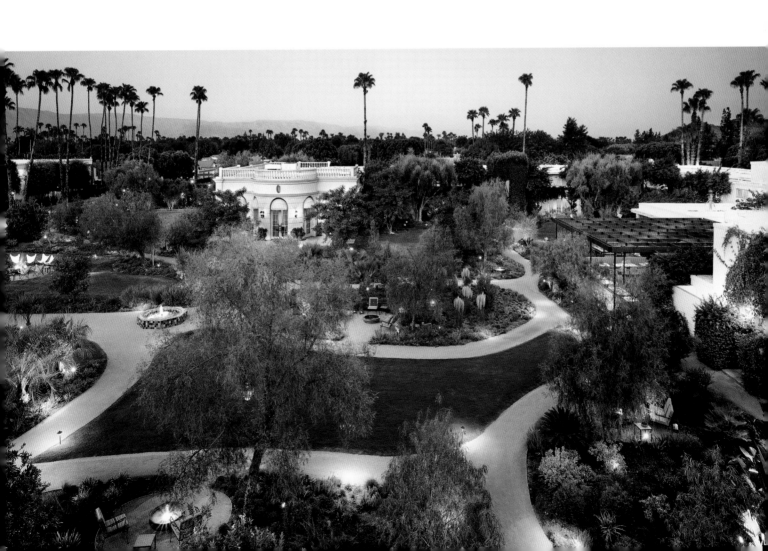

A SELECTED
BIBLIOGRAPHY

HEALING AESTHETICS

Balch, Phyllis A. *Prescription for Herbal Healing*. New York: Avery/Penguin, 2002.

Burnham, Linda. *The Natural Face-Lift*. New York: Barron's Educational Series, Hauppauge, 2003.

Carper, Jean. *Stop Aging Now!: Ultimate Plan for Staying Young and Reversing the Aging Process*. New York: HarperPerennial, 1996.

Carper, Jean. *Miracle Cures: Dramatic New Scientific Discoveries Revealing the Healing Powers of Herbs, Vitamins, and Other Natural Remedies*. New York: HarperPerennial, 1998.

Cohen, Ken. *Honoring the Medicine: The Essential Guide to Native American Healing*. New York: Ballantine Books, 2006.

DuPriest, Laura. *Natural Beauty: Pamper Yourself with Salon Secrets at Home*. Riseville, CA: Prima Publishing, 2002.

Fairley, Josephine. *The Ultimate Natural Beauty Guide*. New York: Universe Publishing, 2004.

Frawley, David. *Ayurvedic Healing: A Comprehensive Guide*, 2nd ed. Twin Lakes, WI: Lotus Press, 2000.

James, Kat. *The Truth About Beauty: Transform Your Looks and Your Life from the Inside Out*. Hillsboro, Oregon: Beyond Words Publishing, Inc., 2003.

Kuczynski, Alex. *Beauty Junkies: Inside Our $15 Billion Obsession with Cosmetic Surgery*. New York: Doubleday, 2006.

Kurz, Susan West, with Tom Monte. *Awakening Beauty the Dr. Hauschka Way*. New York: Clarkson Potter, 2006.

Lad, Vasant. *Ayurveda: The Science of Self-Healing*. Twin Lakes, WI: Lotus Press, 1985.

Manniche, Lise. *Sacred Luxuries: Fragrance, Aromatherapy, and Cosmetics in Ancient Egypt*. Ithaca, NY: Cornell University Press, 1999.

Morrison, Judith H. *The Book of Ayurveda: An Interactive Guide to Using Indian Healing for Personal Wellbeing*. London: Gaia Books Limited, 1994.

Raichur, Pratima, with Marian Cohn. *Absolute Beauty*. New York: HarperCollins, 1997.

Rosas, Debbie and Carlos. *The Nia Technique: The High-Powered Energizing Workout that Gives You a New Body and a New Life*. New York: Broadway Books, 2005.

Sachs, Melanie. *Ayurvedic Beauty Care*. Twin Lakes, WI: Lotus Press, 1994.

Tyldesley, Joyce. *Daughters of Isis: Women of Ancient Egypt*. London: Penguin Books, 1995.

Vukovic, Laurel. *Herbal Healing Secrets for Women*. New York: Prentice Hall, 2000.

Weil, Andrew. *Health and Healing: The Philosophy of Integrative Medicine and Optimum Health*. New York: Houghton Mifflin, 2004.

Weil, Andrew. *Healthy Aging: A Lifelong Guide to Your Physical and Spiritual Well-Being*. New York: Knopf, 2005.

FOOD AND EATING FOR RADIANT HEALTH

Balch, Phyllis A. *Prescription for Dietary Wellness*, 2nd ed. New York: Avery/Penguin, 2003.

Baroody, Theodore A. *Alkalize or Die*. Waynesville, NC: Holographic Health Press, 1991.

Bieler, Henry G. *Food Is Your Best Medicine*. New York: Random House, 1965.

Carper, Jean. *Food—Your Miracle Medicine*. New York: HarperPerennial, 1994.

Chopra, Deepak, David Simon, and Leanne Backer. *The Chopra Center Cookbook: A Nutritional Guide to Renewal/Nourishing Body and Soul*. New York: John Wiley & Sons, 2003.

Colbin, Annemarie. *Food and Healing*. New York: Ballantine Books, 1986.

Colbin, Annemarie. *The Book of Whole Meals*. New York: Ballantine Books, 1985.

Cool, Jesse Ziff. *Your Organic Kitchen: The Essential Guide to Selecting and Cooking Organic Foods*. Emmaus, PA: Rodale Press, 2002.

Frawley, David and Subhash Ranade. *Ayurveda, Nature's Medicine*. Twin Lakes, WI: Lotus Press, 2001.

Fuhrman, Joel, M.D., *Eat to Live*. New York: Little, Brown, and Co., 2003.

Lad, Usha, and Dr. Vasant Lad. *Ayurvedic Cooking for Self-Healing*, 2nd ed. Albuquerque: The Ayurvedic Press, 2002.

Light, Luise. *What To Eat: The Ten Things You Really Need to Know to Eat Well and Be Healthy!* New York: McGraw-Hill, 2005.

Luard, Elisabeth. *Sacred Foods: Cooking for Spiritual Nourishment*. Chicago: Chicago Review Press, Inc., 2001.

Meyerowitz, Steve. *The Organic Food Guide: How to Shop Smarter and Eat Healthier*. Guilford, CT: Globe Pequot Press, 2004.

Mitchell, Paulette. *The 15-Minute Gourmet: Chicken*. New York: John Wiley & Sons, 1999.

Mitchell, Paulette. *The 15-Minute Gourmet: Vegetarian*. New York: John Wiley & Sons, 2000.

Murray, Michael, and Joseph Pizzorno. *The Encyclopedia of Healing Foods*. New York: Atria Books, 2005.

Newman, Nell, with Joseph D'Agnese. *The Newman's Own Organics Guide to a Good Life*. New York: Villard, 2003.

Nienstadt, Yvonne. *Cal-a-Vie's Gourmet Spa Cookery*. Self-published by Cal-a-Vie, 1997.

Ornish, Dean. *Dr. Dean Ornish's Program for Reversing Heart Disease*. New York: Ballantine Books, 1996.

Ornish, Dean. *Eat More, Weigh Less: Dr. Dean Ornish's Life Choice Program for Losing Weight Safely While Eating Abundantly*. New York: HarperCollins, 1993.

Pitchford, Paul. *Healing with Whole Foods: Asian Traditions and Modern Nutrition*, 3rd ed. Berkeley, California: North Atlantic Books, 2002.

Pruess, Joanna with John Harney. *Tea Cuisine: A New Approach to Flavoring Contemporary and Traditional Dishes*. Guilford, Connecticut: The Lyons Press/The Globe Pequot Press, 2006.

Rubin, Jordan S., and Joseph Brasco. *Restoring Your Digestive Health*. New York: Kensington Publishing, 2003.

Stroot, Michel. *The Golden Door Cooks Light & Easy*. Layton, Utah: Gibbs Smith, Publisher, 2003.

Young, Robert O., and Shelley Redford Young. *The pH Miracle: Balance Your Diet, Reclaim Your Health*. New York: Warner Books, 2002.

THE MEDITATIVE ARTS AND SPIRITUAL WELL-BEING

Chinmoy, Sri. *Wings of Joy*. New York: Fireside/Simon and Schuster, 1997.

Chinmoy, Sri. *Meditation: Man-Perfection in God-Satisfaction*. New York: Aum Publications, 1989.

Messervy, Julie M. *The Inward Garden: Creating a Place of Beauty and Meaning*. New York: Little, Brown and Company, 1995.

Ornish, Dean. *Love and Survival*. New York: HarperCollins Publishers, 1998.

Sorin, Fran. *Digging Deep: Unearthing Your Creative Roots Through Gardening*. New York: 2004.

SPAS, BATHS, AND WATERS

Altman, Nathaniel. *Healing Springs: The Ultimate Guide to Taking the Waters*. Rochester, Vermont: Healing Arts Press, 2000.

Altman, Nathaniel. *Sacred Water: The Spiritual Source of Life*. Mahwah, New Jersey: Hidden Spring, 2002.

Batamenghelidj, Fereydoon. *Your Body's Many Cries for Water*. Vienna: Global Health Solutions, Inc., 1997.

Croutier, Alev Lytle. *Taking the Waters: Spirit, Art, Sensuality*. New York: Abbeville Press, 1992.

De Bonneville, Francoise. *The Book of the Bath*. Translated by Jane Brenton. New York: Rizzoli International, 1998.

Emoto, Masaru. *The Hidden Messages in Water*. Translated by David A. Thayne Hillsboro, Oregon: Beyond Words Publishing, 2004.

Emoto, Masaru. *The True Power of Water*. Translated by Noriko Hoysoyamada. Hillsboro, Oregon: Beyond Words Publishing, 2005.

Meyerowitz, Steve. *Water: The Ultimate Cure*. Barrington, MA: Sproutman Publications, 2001.

Seki, Akihiko, and Elizabeth H. Brooke. *The Japanese Spa*. Ruthland, Vermont: Tuttle Publishing, 2005.

Smith, Bruce, and Yoshiko Yamamoto. *The Japanese Bath*. Layton, Utah: Gibbs Smith, Publisher, 2001.

Strausfogel, Sherrie, and Sophia V. Schweitzer. *Hawaii's Spa Experience*. Honolulu: Mutual Publishing, 2004.

Valenza, Janet Mace. *Taking the Waters in Texas: Springs, Spas, and Fountains of Youth*. Austin: University of Texas Press, 2000.

Young, Stanley. *Beautiful Spas and Hot Springs of California*. San Francisco: Chronicle Books, 1998.

The dramatic foyer at the Palm Springs Parker Meridien Spa in California. (Courtesy photo)

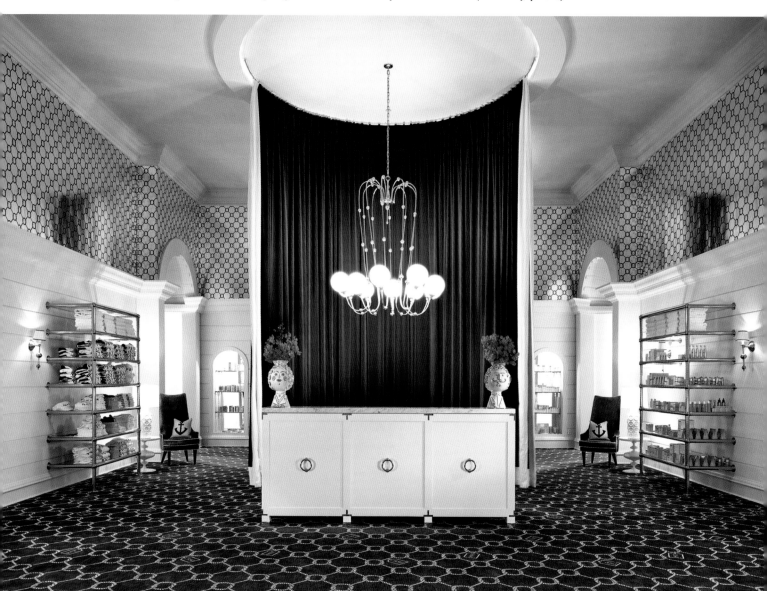

PHOTOGRAPHY CREDITS

The principal photographer for this book is Kim Kurian.

Courtesy photography from the following day spas:
La Posada de Santa Fe Resort & Avanyu Spa, Santa Fe, New Mexico
BODY Café & Spa, Santa Fe, New Mexico
Chopra Dream Center New York
Cornelia Day Spa & Resort, New York
El Monte Sagrado, Taos, New Mexico
Four Seasons Hotel, Philadelphia
Four Seasons Hotel, New York City
Four Seasons Hotel Washington, D.C.
Ihilani Resort & Spa, Oahu, Hawaii
Mandarin Oriental, New York
Nob Hill Spa at The Huntington Hotel, San Francisco
Ojo Caliente Hot Springs and Spa, New Mexico
Parker Meridien Resort & Spa, New York City
Parker Meridien Resort & Spa, Palm Springs, California
SpaHalekulani, Honolulu
SpaOlakino, Honolulu
Spa Vitale, San Francisco
Tamaya Mist Spa & Salon, Albuquerque, New Mexico
Terme di Aroma, Philadelphia
The Westin at Times Square, New York City

Courtesy photography from the following destination spas:
Cal-a-Vie, Vista, California
Golden Door, Escondido, California
Rancho La Puerta, Baja California, Mexico

INDEX